The

Psoas

Solution

The practitioner's guide to rehabilitation, corrective exercise, and training for improved function

Evan Osar

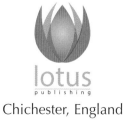

lotus
publishing

Chichester, England

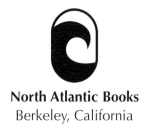

North Atlantic Books

Berkeley, California

First published in 2017 by
Lotus Publishing
Apple Tree Cottage, Inlands Road, Nutbourne, Chichester, PO18 8RJ and
North Atlantic Books
Berkeley, California

All Drawings Amanda Williams, Matt Lambert
Photographs on pages 23, 47, 51, 65, 68, 93, 94, 103, 126, 129, 142, 143, 144, 150, 154, 178, 180, and 196 supplied courtesy of shutterstock. All other photographs supplied by the author unless otherwise indicated.
Cover and Text Design by Medlar Publishing Solutions Pvt Ltd, India
Printed and Bound in the UK by Bell & Bain Limited

The Psoas Solution: The Practitioner's Guide to Rehabilitation, Corrective Exercise, and Training for Improved Function is sponsored and published by the Society for the Study of Native Arts and Sciences (dba North Atlantic Books), an educational nonprofit based in Berkeley, California, that collaborates with partners to develop cross-cultural perspectives, nurture holistic views of art, science, the humanities, and healing, and seed personal and global transformation by publishing work on the relationship of body, spirit, and nature.

North Atlantic Books' publications are available through most bookstores. For further information, visit our website at www.northatlanticbooks.com or call 800-733-3000.

British Library Cataloguing-in-Publication Data
A CIP record for this book is available from the British Library
ISBN 978 1 905367 78 8 (Lotus Publishing)
ISBN 978 1 62317 135 3 (North Atlantic Books)

Library of Congress Cataloging-in-Publication Data
Names: Osar, Evan, 1969- author.
Title: The psoas solution : the practitioner's guide to rehabilitation, corrective exercise, and training for improved function / Evan Osar.
Description: Berkeley, California : North Atlantic Books, 2017. | Includes bibliographical references.
Identifiers: LCCN 2017005060 (print) | LCCN 2017005665 (ebook) | ISBN 9781623171353 (pbk.) | ISBN 9781623171353 (ebook)
Subjects: | MESH: Physical Therapy Modalities | Psoas Muscles
Classification: LCC QP301 (print) | LCC QP301 (ebook) | NLM WB 460 | DDC 612/.04--dc23
LC record available at https://lccn.loc.gov/2017005060

Contents

This book is dedicated to all the wonderful individuals who have provided me with the opportunity to experiment, discover, and most importantly learn. Thank you for entrusting me with your health.

Acknowledgments

I would like to thank:

My publisher Jon—you are a joy to work with and I am blessed to have a professional relationship with you. Thank you for providing me with the opportunities, as well as the creative freedom, to write and convey my message.

Gretchen—I don't think it was your intention to become my coach after constructively critiquing my first book; this came to be, however, through the process of helping me organize my many scattered thoughts and ideas and articulate them in a way that hopefully helps to educate and empower others. Thank you, Gretchen, for all your guidance, the gentle (and at times not so gentle) encouragement, and the unyielding support over the past few years. My writing and teaching are forever changed because of our work together.

My incredibly loving and supportive wife Jenice— you give me the support, you provide me with a foundation, and every day you challenge me to be the best that I can be. I am blessed every single day of my life because you are a part of it.

I believe humility is essential to continued learning and growing. If one regards oneself as smarter or more knowledgeable than everyone else, one will lack the incentive to seek out and learn from the smartest people in one's chosen field. I want to recognize and thank a few of the many brilliant individuals I have had the honor of studying with and learning from over the years. These individuals are some of the true geniuses in the industry, and in learning from them, I am constantly reminded of the famous quote from Sir Isaac Newton: "If I have seen further it is by standing on the shoulders of giants." Although by no means exhaustive, my list of such individuals includes: Dr. Linda-Joy Lee, Diane Lee, Shirley Sahrmann, Karel Lewit, Vladimir Janda, Pavel Kolar, and the Prague School instructors, Dr. Paul Hodges, Gwendolyn Jull, Carol Richardson, Julie Hides, and Sean Gibbons. Having the opportunity to learn from these individuals keeps me humble. Their contributions can be seen throughout the book.

Evan Osar

Preface

If you purchased or were given *The Psoas Solution* as a gift, you likely fall into one of two categories:

1. You are a chiropractic physician, medical doctor, physical therapist, fitness professional, or manual therapist who works with individuals experiencing low back, pelvis, and/or hip issues that you suspect are related to their psoas.

   I hope this resource increases your current base of knowledge and, more importantly, provides you with some practical information that can assist you in working with your clients or patients who are experiencing chronic postural and movement syndromes related to their psoas as well as with those individuals who want to continue functioning at a high level.

2. You are someone experiencing chronic low back or pelvic or hip problems and have been told by your chiropractic physician, medical doctor, physical therapist, fitness professional, or massage therapist that your psoas is the cause of your issue.

   I hope you find this book helpful. However, while I utilize with my own patients all the techniques and strategies it presents, *unfortunately I cannot guarantee that the solution to your unique issue lies within the covers of this book. Your health care practitioner can determine whether or not the information it contains is applicable to your situation. If it is, and if you are diligent and patient in the process and use the information that is appropriate to your unique situation, I hope this resource can assist you in developing more optimal posture and movement habits.*

About The Psoas Solution

This book represents a compilation of the information currently available on the psoas, blended with clinical evidence and integrated with practical applications of the concepts. It is not intended to provide quick-fix solutions to your own or your client's/patient's postural or movement dysfunctions, or to chronic low back, pelvis, and/or spine issues. As with life itself, the development of a more optimal posture or movement strategy, or the improvement of one's chronic issues, is a journey rather than a destination. The solution lies in the journey, in the self-discovery of one's habits, and in the identification of more effective strategies for expressing optimal posture and movement. While this journey often ends in a successful outcome, it does not always result in the achievement of one's health and fitness goals, or in a complete resolution of one's tightness, pain, or dysfunction.

One's successes—as well as one's failures—in improving posture, movement, and overall health often mirror one's life; they are the result of an intricate and interwoven set of factors. In other words, optimal health and function are often a combination of many factors and are not always related to what they appear to be associated with on the surface.

A person's posture and movement strategy, as well as the non-optimal habits contributing to their musculoskeletal dysfunction, are invariably linked to multiple factors, including (but not limited to) medical history, occupation, activity level, rest, recuperation, exercise (or lack of), nutrition, and genetics. Similarly, they are impacted by a variety of psychosocial factors, including emotions, motivation, purpose, beliefs, and the presence or absence of a support system. It is beyond the scope of this book to comprehensively identify what is ultimately driving a person's issues—physical, physiological, or psychological—or what is preventing them from accomplishing a personal health or fitness goal, and then determine who is the best professional for them to work with.

The goals of *The Psoas Solution* are threefold:

1. To help you discover and appreciate the functional anatomy of the psoas and its relationship to posture and movement.

2. To identify and discuss the common signs associated with the non-optimal use of the psoas in posture and movement.

3. To develop a system-based corrective and progressive exercise approach that integrates the three key principles related to the development and maintenance of optimal posture and movement.

If you are a health/fitness professional, you will likely discover something within this book—and hopefully several things—that will help your clients or patients achieve a positive outcome. By understanding and applying the concepts and principles that will be discussed in this book, and integrating them into your current approach with which you have already had success, you will undoubtedly help many individuals apply a more optimal posture and movement strategy so that they can achieve their health and fitness goals.

If you personally have been told or suspect that you have a problem with your psoas, and you have either been given this book as a gift or picked it up in the hope it will help you, it is important that you recognize the information contained within requires at least a basic knowledge of anatomy and exercise. Do not attempt any exercise without first clearing it with your own health care professional, so that you know the information is appropriate and applicable to your unique situation. I hope that this book supports you on your journey to achieving your personal health and fitness goals.

Onward …

Abbreviations

APT	anterior pelvic tilt (rotation)	ITB	iliotibial band
ASIS	anterior superior iliac spine	IMS™	Integrative Movement System™
CES	corrective exercise strategy	LBP	low back pain
DDD	degenerative disc disease	PMj	psoas major
DJD	degenerative joint disease	PMn	psoas minor
DMS	deep myofascial system	PPT	posterior pelvic tilt (rotation)
EMG	electromyography	PSIS	posterior superior iliac spine
FAI	femoroacetabular impingement	SMS	superficial myofascial system
FPR	frontal plane rotation	SPR	sagittal plane rotation
GERD	gastroesophageal reflux disease	TFL	tensor fasciae latae
GMax	gluteus maximus	TLJ	thoracolumbar junction
GMin	gluteus minimus	TPC	thoracopelvic cylinder
GMed	gluteus medius	TPR	transverse plane rotation

Introduction

I remember it as clearly as if it happened just yesterday. It was about 18 years ago, early in my first year or two of practice. I was working with a significant number of Chicago's professional dancers during my first job out of chiropractic school—members of Hubbard Street Dance Chicago, Joffrey Ballet Company, and several smaller professional dance companies. A requirement for powerful and beautiful dance is full range—and oftentimes excessive range—of hip extension to achieve positions such as arabesque and grand battement. And when I asked the dancer presenting for work what area they would most like me to focus on during that session, the hip flexors would unequivocally be the most common area in which they complained of tightness and where they needed greater flexibility.

In school I had learned about the *lower crossed syndrome*—a posture characterized by excessive anterior pelvic tilt and increased lumbar lordosis. This concept was reinforced in almost every article I read on low back pain, as well as in continuing education courses I attended. I would perform my assessments as I had been taught in school and at my continuing education workshops; when I carried out a postural assessment, I noticed anterior pelvic tilt and hyperlordosis on every single dancer I saw.

I confidently believed that I had the solution to these dancer's hip problems: stretch the hip flexors (especially the psoas, since this was the muscle that I learned was most responsible for anterior hip tightness) and strengthen the glutes. After all, this is what I had learned to be the "Holy Grail solution" to the lower crossed syndrome and most causes of low back pain. However, when I performed the Modified Thomas Test (see Appendix I: Assessing the Psoas), I often got mixed information. During the Modified Thomas Test, you would expect to see a shortened psoas if the individual has an anterior pelvic tilt and hyperlordotic curve in their lumbar spine. However, this is not what I was finding: contrary to what I had learned, nearly every dancer I evaluated had what appeared to be an *overlengthened* psoas.

Not having enough clinical experience to rely on, and putting far too much trust in my postural evaluation and the dancer's self-assessment of feeling "really tight" in their hip flexors, I assumed I was missing something and obliged them by continuing to stretch the psoas and other hip flexors. Additionally, I would have them perform gluteus maximus exercises to strengthen the "weak" and "inhibited" antagonist to the psoas. As far as I could determine at the time, I had mixed success with this approach. Some dancers would feel great afterwards and want more of that approach; others, however, would mention increased tightness in their posterior hip and low back. I chalked this up to the fact that we probably had not stretched or strengthened enough and that they likely needed a follow-up visit or two.

Unfortunately, I used this strategy one day on a dancer with chronic hip tightness and low back discomfort, and she experienced increased low back discomfort following the treatment. She was unable to dance that evening, and it took several weeks of therapy to get her back to dancing. Needless to say, she was not very confident in my services after that. In my private practice, more and more patients were beginning to relate similar stories. I can recall cases of two different patients around the same time who "threw" their backs out after leaving my session during which I had stretched their psoas and had them working on strengthening their abdominals and glutes. This was not what I had learned was supposed to happen following this tried-and-true protocol.

Looking back now, I can clearly see what the problem was; I was only seeing what I had been trained to see. As Ralph Waldo Emerson said: "People only see what they are prepared to see." Now I can look back and recognize that I was not seeing a true anterior pelvic tilt and lumbar hyperlordosis—I had been trained to look for it and that is why I saw it. (Note: this book will discuss what I was truly seeing in these dancers and in many of my patients and how so many individuals are actually presenting quite differently from what many of us have been taught.)

Furthermore, I was trying to fit every individual—and I stress the word *individual*—into a treatment protocol, rather than really understanding what I was seeing (overlengthened psoas and hip flexors) in my dancers and patients and addressing it appropriately.

As the famous quote attributed to Mark Twain suggests, I had let my education get in the way of my learning. Had I heard this quote—and more importantly actually understood what it meant—I would have taken a very different approach with the dancers and patients who I was treating so many years ago. However, nothing really replaces the importance of clinical or practical experience … except, perhaps, the lessons that one must learn from these experiences. Truth be told, the concept of the increased anterior pelvic tilt and lumbar lordosis causing low back and hip issues, as well as a host of other dysfunctions, is as pervasive in rehabilitation and training environments today as it was so many years ago.

Since those early self-deprecating days in practice, and wondering if I would ever be good enough or know enough to actually help anyone, I have approached my work with a much more open mind and with much greater humility. I am constantly evaluating, treating and/or training, and re-evaluating every single one of the individuals who entrust me with their care. And while I am happy that I am able to help many of them achieve their health and fitness goals, I am much more interested in the ones I am not able to help—those individuals who, I feel, should be improving and are doing the necessary work to improve, yet are still experiencing chronic dysfunction that inhibits them from achieving their health and fitness goals.

We are validated by our successes, but we learn from our failures. Every single day that I am in practice is a day of learning. Each day I am validated … and each day I am presented with opportunities for continued learning. When I fail to help a patient achieve their goals, I embark on a new path of discovery and learning.

This book is really a "clinical snapshot" of the lessons I have learned throughout my years in practice, working with thousands of individuals with dysfunctions of the low back, pelvis, and hip. For lack of a better term, it is also a compendium of the approaches we use in our clinic on ordinary people—not just on the athletes and high-performing individuals—with back, pelvic, and hip dysfunctions.

How is this book organized and how can it help you? This book is designed to tell a story about the psoas, with each chapter building upon the information developed in previous chapters. Nevertheless, each chapter contains enough practical information so that if you want to jump ahead you can still find the information applicable to the respective chapter topic. If you find yourself jumping ahead and have questions regarding the exercises, be sure to go back and read the earlier chapters, in particular Chapter 1 on the functional anatomy, so that you can fill in any gaps that might arise in later sections.

As mentioned above, Chapter 1 will cover functional anatomy, i.e. the bony and fascial attachments of the psoas, and on the basis of this architecture what this muscle most likely does in terms of function (posture and movement). Several commonly held beliefs about the psoas will be addressed in this first chapter. For example, if the psoas is purely a hip flexor, why does it attach to every vertebral level from T11 through L5, and why does it fascially blend into the diaphragm, transversus abdominis, and pelvic floor? If the psoas has a role in the motion of the pelvis, what do the attachments to the front of the pelvis suggest that the muscle's impact on pelvic motion truly is? On the basis of its anatomy and the available clinical research to date, I will propose that the psoas' function is far more diverse than that of a simple hip flexor, and argue against its contribution to the anterior tilt posture. Additionally, I will briefly discuss how psoas function is synergistically related to several muscles of the trunk, spine, pelvis, and

hip complex, including the multifidi, iliacus, and gluteus maximus.

There is an ongoing debate regarding the concept of core stabilization and its contribution to both spinal stabilization and overall performance. This debate does not center so much on whether or not core stability is important, but on which muscles are most important and which strategy is most effective in providing ideal core stability. While often disregarded in the discussion, three-dimensional breathing is an important component of developing and maintaining an optimal core stabilization strategy. In Chapter 2 I will discuss the concept of three-dimensional breathing and the role the psoas plays in stabilizing the trunk, spine, and pelvis during respiration. There is no research that discusses the role of the psoas and breathing, but given its fascial connections to the diaphragm and pelvic floor I take the liberty of suggesting that the psoas likely has an important role both in breathing and in core stability.

Chapter 3 will introduce how to develop an efficient core and hip stabilization strategy based upon the latest research on the topic, as well as providing examples of how we can incorporate these concepts into our own patients' programs.

Ultimately, the key to successfully improving psoas function lies in the ability to incorporate the use of this muscle in the fundamental movement patterns. The fundamental movement patterns are those patterns that are essential to most activities in life. In essence, most of our activities of daily life, sport, and occupation can be broken down into seven fundamental movements. In Chapters 4–7 I introduce a few of the fundamental movement patterns and discuss the psoas' involvement in them. While this list of movement patterns is not exhaustive, I will discuss the psoas' involvement in squatting, lunging, bending, and hip flexion/extension patterns. Again, where there is no current research to suggest the psoas' role, I will extrapolate its function on the basis of the previous functional anatomy discussion, so that we will at least have a place to begin the discussion of the muscle's contribution during movement.

In the conclusion I will discuss our current knowledge limitations and where additional research into the psoas will be beneficial.

I have also included several additional topics relating to the psoas in the appendices at the end of the book; these appendices are designed to address some common topics related to the psoas that were not dealt with in the chapters. The appendices contain discussions of posture; assessment; the role of corrective exercise; sitting posture for ensuring optimal psoas function; the relationship between the pelvic floor and the psoas; and the psoas' involvement in common hip pathologies, such as labral tears and femoroacetabular impingement (FAI).

Which strategy is the *best* one for enhancing psoas function and ultimately improving posture and movement? Unfortunately, that is not an easy question to answer and was not my goal in writing this book. It is not my intention that this book become the "gold standard" for improving psoas function and/or for invalidating previous information and clinical approaches that have been applied with success to the psoas. It is instead an attempt to expand the conversation as well as to share what I have observed in clinical practice, along with the strategies that my team at Chicago Integrative Movement Specialists have been implementing over the past dozen or so years to improve posture and more importantly, movement efficiency in our patients and clients.

It is my hope that this book will make you think and help broaden your perspective about how the psoas contributes to achieving and maintaining optimal posture and movement.

Before we begin, I would like to make one final point for health and fitness professionals: continue to do what you have been successful with. If you have a unique way of working with individuals with psoas issues and have had success, then continue to use those techniques and strategies. Let this book serve as a guide for you and to help you consider things you may have not thought about, or as an adjunct to your current treatment/ training program with which you are already having success.

Online Video Content

To access the online video content:

1. Visit the website www.IIHFE.com/the-psoas-solution.
2. You will be directed to **Sign Up** to gain access to the video content.
3. Once you have provided your information, you will be granted immediate access.

The following video content is available online:

- Three-dimensional Breathing
  - Apical to pelvis (top to bottom)
  - Lateral or costal (side to side)
  - Antero-posterior (front to back)
- Thoracopelvic Cylinder and Hip Stabilization
  - Happy Baby Unsupported
  - Happy Baby with Dumbbell Pull-over
  - Happy Baby with Heel Drop
- Squat
  - Supported
  - Parallel
  - Split
- Lunge
  - Forward
  - Reverse
  - Elevated rear leg
- Bending
  - Spinal flexion
    - Forward Bending
    - Pelvic Tilt

- Hip Hinge
  - Supported
  - Unsupported
- Spine and Hip Extension
  - Spine Extension
    - Prone Lengthen
    - Back Bending
  - Bird Dog
  - Hip Hinge Bridge
  - Marching Bridge
  - Single-leg Bridge

- Psoas Assessment
  - Modified Thomas Test
  - Impingement Test
  - Manual Muscle Test
- Neutral Alignment
  - Standing Assessment
  - Pelvic alignment and motion
- Suspension
- Sitting Posture

Diagram of Body Image

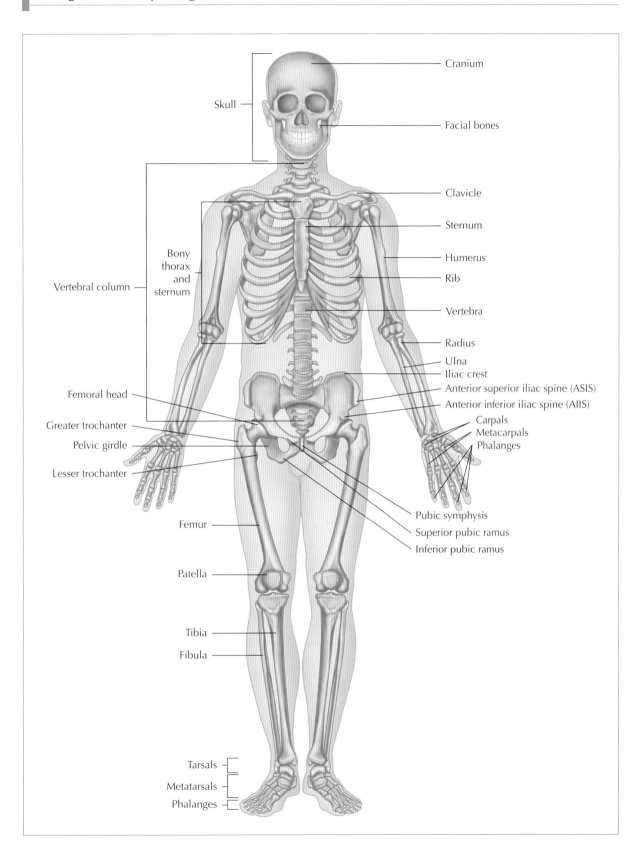

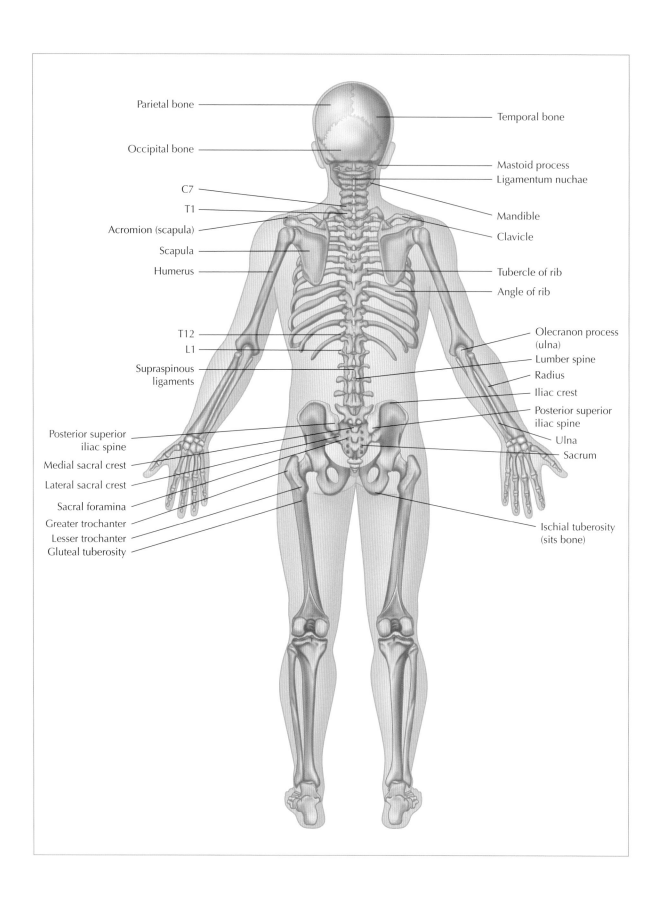

Parietal bone

Temporal bone

Occipital bone

Mastoid process

Ligamentum nuchae

C7

T1

Mandible

Acromion (scapula)

Clavicle

Scapula

Humerus

Tubercle of rib

Angle of rib

T12

Olecranon process
(ulna)

L1

Lumber spine

Supraspinous
ligaments

Radius

Iliac crest

Posterior superior
iliac spine

Posterior superior
iliac spine

Ulna

Medial sacral crest

Sacrum

Lateral sacral crest

Sacral foramina

Greater trochanter

Lesser trochanter

Ischial tuberosity
(sits bone)

Gluteal tuberosity

Functional Anatomy of the Psoas

Perhaps no muscle in the body that invites the attention of students, chiropractic physicians, physical therapists, medical doctors, and fitness professionals is more misunderstood or maligned than the psoas. It is commonly blamed for causing a multitude of musculoskeletal problems, including low back pain, hip tightness, and gluteal inhibition. It is further disparaged because it is associated with being the primary muscle responsible for contributing to common postural dysfunctions, including anterior pelvic tilt and excessive lumbar lordosis. The psoas is surgically released when thought to be contributing to impingement, labral, and "snapping" issues related to the hip (Hwang et al. 2015, Dobbs et al. 2002, Taylor and Clark 1995).

To gain an understanding and appreciation of how the psoas is really functioning in posture and movement, this chapter will explore the functional anatomy of the muscle in terms of where it attaches and its impact upon the related joints. Although interest and research is on the increase, the overall knowledge of the actual function of the psoas is somewhat lacking compared with other muscles; however, evidence-based information about its function, where available, will be provided. Where information is not available, a combination of related research and clinical experience will be used to extrapolate, and either expand upon or dispute, the commonly accepted knowledge of the psoas.

Psoas Attachments

Theoretically, the psoas assists in stabilizing the central rod (spine) within the thoracopelvic cylinder (TPC) (Osar 2015). The fascial attachments connecting the psoas from the diaphragm to the pelvic floor and into the pelvis suggest that, in addition to its impact on the hip, the psoas has a global role in the stability of the lower portion of the TPC.

The psoas major (PMj) originates from the anterior lateral surfaces of the vertebral bodies and transverse processes of each vertebra from level T12 through L5. It also attaches to the intervertebral discs of the lumbar spine, apart from L5–S1. Superiorly, the fascia of the psoas blends into the crura of the diaphragm and is continuous with the transversus abdominis (Stecco 2015, Gibbons 2005ab, Gibbons 2007, Myers 2014). The fascia covering the posterior diaphragm connects the diaphragm, quadratus lumborum, and psoas (Bordoni and Zanier 2013).

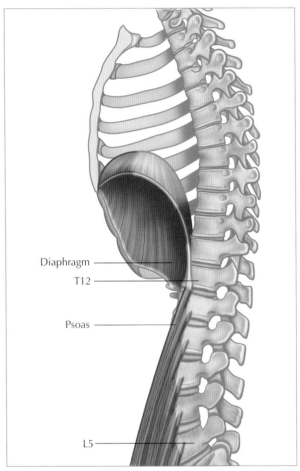

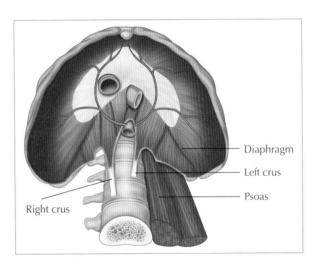

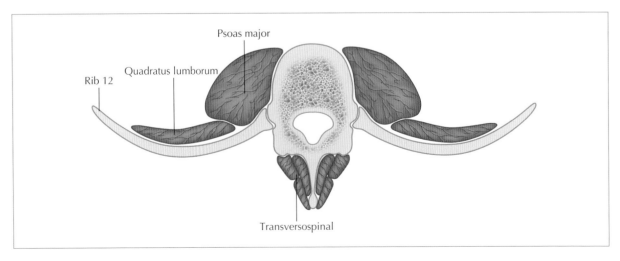

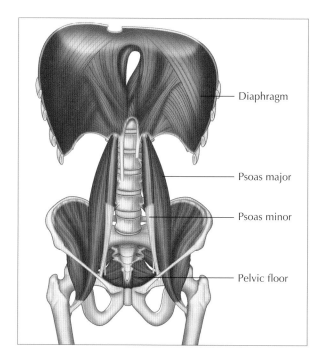

Diaphragm

Psoas major

Psoas minor

Pelvic floor

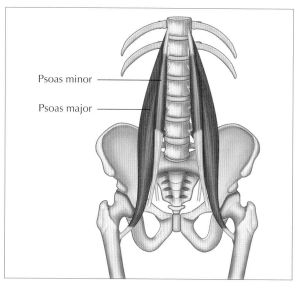

Psoas minor

Psoas major

Distally, the PMj becomes thickened, blending into the pelvic floor and fascially integrating with the lower fibers of the transversus abdominis and internal oblique muscles (Gibbons 2005ab, Gibbons 2007). It attaches to the pelvic brim, as well as fascially blending into the pelvic floor, before passing inferiorly to insert into the lesser trochanter of the femur (Gibbons 2005ab, Gibbons 2007). Thus, the psoas functions as a myofascial connection between the diaphragm and the pelvic floor (image above).

It has been reported that 40–50% of the population do not have a psoas minor (PMn) muscle (Stecco 2015, Myers 2014, Franklin 2011, FitzGordon 2013), although it was present in 65.6% of the 32 hips dissected by Neumann and Garceau (2014). When present, the PMn originates from the lower two thoracic vertebrae, adjoining ribs, and intervertebral discs, and inserts into the superior ramus of the pelvis. In individuals where the PMn is absent, the PMj sends fibers that blend into the iliac fascia at the iliopectineal eminence (Stecco 2015, Myers 2014).

To better understand the function of the psoas, the next section will focus on motion associated with the spine-pelvis-hip complex.

Joint Motion and Centration

The psoas has a very specific influence on several joints of the body, including the hip, spine, and pelvis. This book will discuss the psoas' role in the control of posture and motion in these regions.

A joint is formed where two bones *articulate*, or join together and allow motion. The size and shape of the joint, as well as the nature of the muscles, fascia, and ligaments surrounding it, determine the amount of motion available at that joint.

A *synovial joint* contains synovial fluid and cartilaginous end surfaces covering each bone of the articulation, and is surrounded by a ligamentous joint capsule. Optimal joint mobility—set up by proper alignment and control—stimulates the production of synovial fluid, while optimal rest (non-weight bearing positions) allows the joints to decompress. Appropriate loading and unloading of synovial joints are key components in promoting and maintaining joint health and longevity. Prolonged compression secondary to myofascial gripping is a common cause of degenerative joint disease.

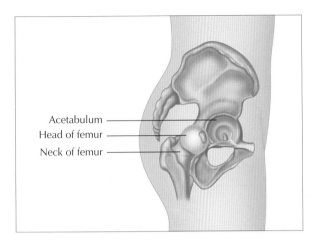

Acetabulum
Head of femur
Neck of femur

The hip joint—formed by the femoral head of the femur articulating with the acetabulum of the pelvis—is a synovial joint (image above). With optimal alignment and control, the joint can withstand normal forces, and hence regular joint aging occurs. With altered alignment and control, and/or myofascial gripping that results in over-compression of the joint, the resulting chronic wear and tear will degenerate the joint, leading to degenerative joint disease.

As well as synovial joints, the spine contains *cartilaginous joints*, which are formed by two bones adjoined to a disc of cartilage. In the spine, two adjacent vertebrae (bones) are connected via an intervertebral disc (cartilaginous disc). The facet joints, which help guide spinal and rib motion, are formed by two adjacent vertebrae and are categorized as synovial joints (image below).

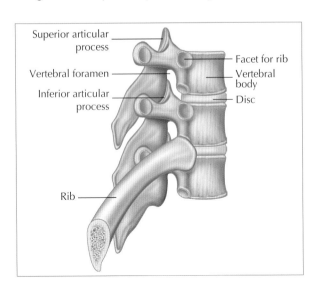

Superior articular process
Vertebral foramen
Inferior articular process
Rib
Facet for rib
Vertebral body
Disc

Joint Motion of the Hips, Spine, and Pelvis

Regardless of the type of joint, its motion is generally named according to what the proximal bone of the articulation (the bone closest to the center of the body) is doing relative to the distal bone (the bone furthest away from the center of the body).

Hip Motion

There are two ways of looking at motion at the hip: 1) what happens when the femur moves relative to the pelvis; and 2) what occurs when the pelvis moves relative to the femur. For example, hip flexion occurs by moving or flexing the femoral head while the pelvis remains stationary. Similarly, the pelvis can rotate over the femoral head. Therefore, two different actions can result in the same relative motion.

Generally, when the femur moves toward the head, and the acetabulum remains relatively stationary, it is considered *hip flexion*. When the pelvis anteriorly rotates over the femoral heads, this is also hip flexion, although it is most often referred to as *anterior pelvic tilt*. Technically speaking, hip flexion is required to produce any movement pattern where the femoral head is rotating in the acetabulum and the thigh is moving toward the trunk.

Hip motion includes:

- *Hip flexion*—the femur flexes relative to the pelvis, or the pelvis anteriorly rotates (in the sagittal plane) relative to the femur.
- *Hip extension*—the femur extends relative to the pelvis, or the pelvis posteriorly rotates (in the sagittal plane) relative to the femur.
- *Hip rotation*—the femur rotates relative to the pelvis, or the pelvis rotates (in the transverse plane) around the femur.
- *Hip abduction*—the femur abducts relative to the pelvis, or the pelvis laterally flexes (in the frontal plane) over the femur.
- *Hip adduction*—the femur adducts relative to the pelvis, or the pelvis laterally flexes (in the frontal plane) over the femur.

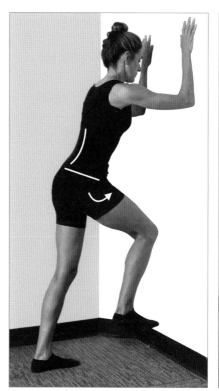 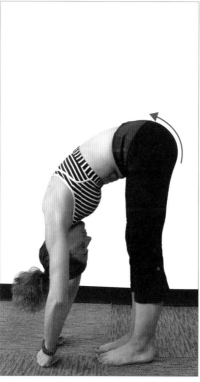 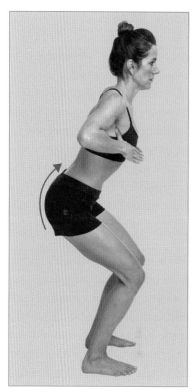

Hip flexion—the femur is moving relative to the pelvis (above left); the pelvis is rotating anteriorly over the femoral heads when bending forward (above middle) and when squatting (above right).

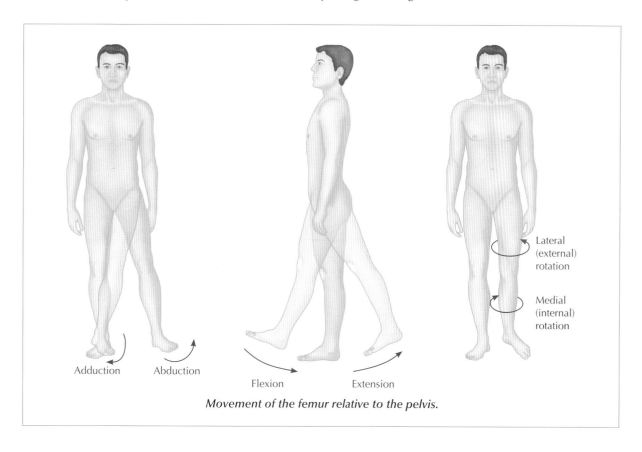

Movement of the femur relative to the pelvis.

Spine Motion

A concept most often related to spinal motion, which will be included in the discussion of bending, is segmental or intersegmental motion (inter = between, segmental = involving segments or vertebrae of the spine). *Segmental* or *intersegmental* motion refers to the movement of one segment, followed by the next segment, followed by the next segment, and so on, with each vertebral segment contributing to the overall motion of the spine.

The ability to segmentally move the spine in any direction is what provides smooth, coordinated, and beautiful movement—in other words, efficient movement. Segmental movement of the spine is what enables an individual the ability to *articulate* their spine or move one segment and then the next, etc. in many exercises (e.g. the Roll-up—see Chapter 6), in a well-executed golf swing, and in activities such as Latin and Hawaiian dance.

Segmental motion of the spine includes:

- *Flexion*—forward bending of the spine in the sagittal plane.
- *Extension*—backward bending of the spine in the sagittal plane.
- *Lateral flexion*—side bending of the spine in the frontal plane.
- *Rotation*—rotation of the spine in the transverse plane.

The inability to move segmentally or articulate through a region (or many regions) of the spine in any of the aforementioned ranges of motion will often overload joints around the restricted area. The *hypomobile* joint segment(s)—a region that is not moving as well as it should—will generally lead to increased motion or *hypermobility* of the surrounding joints, and to the loss of efficient movement.

Degenerative disc disease (DDD) and degenerative joint disease (DJD) generally occur either as a direct result of either prolonged over-compression

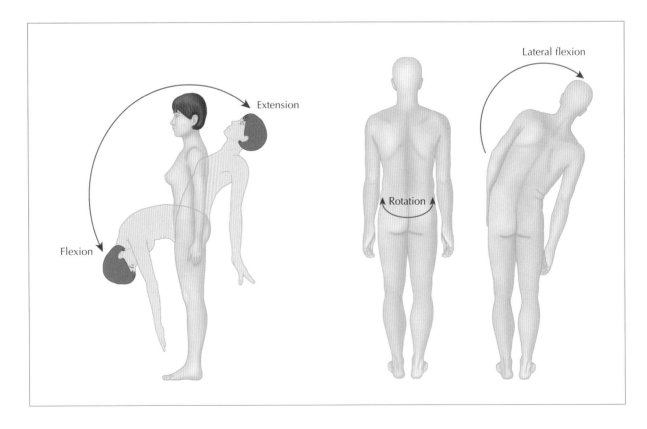

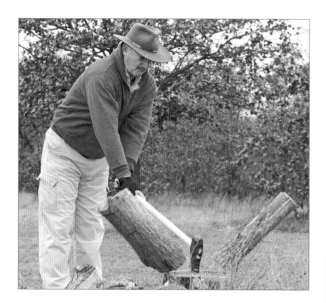

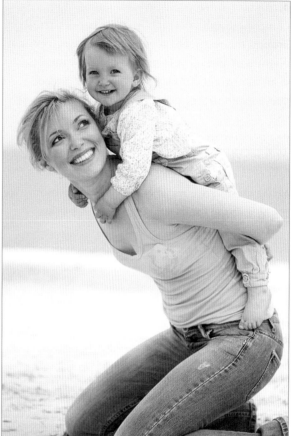

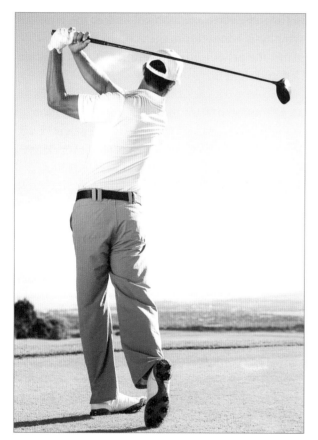

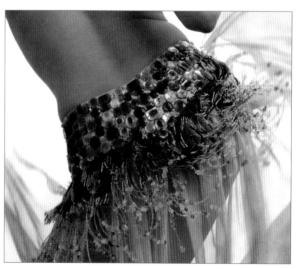

Most activities of life and sport require the ability to move the pelvis over the femoral head while articulating the spine.

secondary to hypomobility or as a result of compensatory hypermobility that has occurred around the restricted segments. Restoring optimal alignment and movement of all joint segments is an important strategy for improving and/or preventing further degenerative changes.

Pelvic Motion

Pelvic motion occurs when the pelvis moves relative to the femoral heads, and is defined as follows:

- *Anterior pelvic tilt*—forward rotation or anterior tilt of the pelvis over the femoral heads. This motion can also be considered hip flexion.
- *Posterior pelvic tilt*—backward rotation or posterior tilt of the pelvis over the femoral heads. This motion can also be considered hip extension.
- *Lateral pelvic tilt*—rotation of the pelvis around the femoral heads in the frontal plane. This motion can also be considered hip abduction on the lower side and hip adduction on the higher side of the pelvic tilt.
- *Transverse plane rotation*—rotation of the pelvis around the femoral heads in the

transverse plane. This motion can also be considered *hip internal rotation* when the pelvis rotates toward one side, and *hip external rotation* on the side away from which the pelvis rotates.

Important consideration regarding pelvic motion:

Pelvic position (pelvis alignment relative to the femoral head) will be determined using the relationship of the ASIS (anterior superior iliac spine) relative to the pubic symphysis. Neutral pelvis—i.e. an anteriorly rotated pelvis (pelvic tilt)—is when the ASIS is slightly anterior to the pubic symphysis in the sagittal plane (middle image below). If the ASIS and pubic symphysis are in the same vertical alignment and/or the pubic symphysis is anterior to the ASIS in the sagittal plane, the pelvis is in a posteriorly rotated position (left and right images below).

More important than the actual resting position of the pelvis is the ability to rotate the pelvis anteriorly over the femoral heads to appropriately flex the hip when performing movements like forward bending, squatting, and hip hinging.

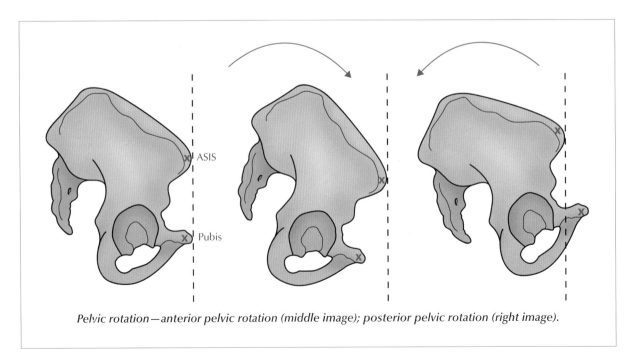

Pelvic rotation—anterior pelvic rotation (middle image); posterior pelvic rotation (right image).

See more on pelvic motion during bending and squatting below.

Forward bending without and with spinal flexion: Beginning from a standing position, the pelvis should anteriorly rotate around the femoral heads during forward bending (a & b). Forward bending in this manner, also referred to as *hip hinging*, optimally loads the posterior hip complex (gluteal complex, hamstrings, calve muscles) and reduces stress upon the lumbar spine; it is the preferred method for lifting heavier objects to, or from the floor, and/or for reducing stress upon the low back. Forward bending with spinal flexion is not a problem for most individuals that don't have spinal issues providing they use their hips appropriately. Note the lack of pelvis motion which results in having to over-flex the spine to make up for the inability to anteriorly rotate the pelvis over the femoral heads

(c). Bending primarily from one's spine with very little contribution from the hips can be a common contributor to chronic low back and pelvic issues. See more on this topic in the bending chapter.

Pelvic rotation (i.e. tilt) during a body weight squat pattern: The starting position of the pelvis (a) is less important than the individual's ability to anteriorly rotate her pelvis (flex the hips) to begin the squat pattern (b & c). Note that the entire thoracopelvic cylinder (TPC) is still connected as she begins the squat pattern meaning this is not an isolated movement of the pelvis. As she descends into the squat pattern she will gradually reverse this position and begin to posteriorly rotate her pelvis while still maintaining overall alignment of her TPC. During the final phase of the pattern, her pelvis continues to rotate posteriorly (c & d).

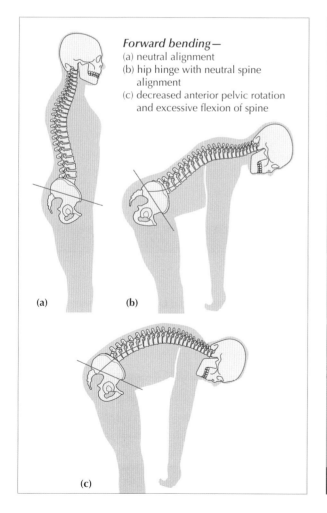

Forward bending—
(a) neutral alignment
(b) hip hinge with neutral spine alignment
(c) decreased anterior pelvic rotation and excessive flexion of spine

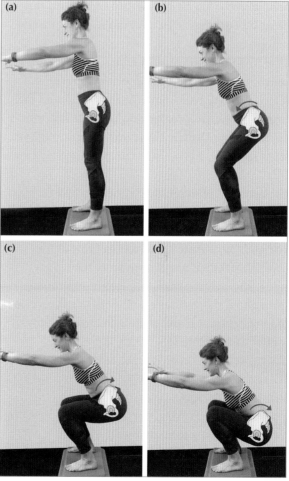

To optimally load the posterior hip complex and reduce stress upon the lumbar spine, it is important that the individual initially starts out anteriorly rotating the pelvis, and as they progress, that they eccentrically control that position through the pattern. This control allows them to continue loading the hips without moving into early or excessive posterior pelvic. See more on topic in the squatting chapter.

Summary: During any pattern that requires hip flexion—sitting, bending forward, squatting, lunging, walking up stairs, deadlifting—the pelvis as part of the thoracopelvic cylinder should anteriorly rotate over the femoral head to optimally position the pelvis and spine and load the posterior hip complex. During body weight squats and/or when bending forward, the spine can relatively flex as part of the movement pattern as long as the individual is still moving their hips. These mechanics support optimal psoas length and control and in turn the psoas is better able to support optimal posture and movement. Low back and pelvic problems tend to arise when the individual overuses spinal flexion to compensate for a tight posterior hip complex and an inability to optimally move their pelvis around their femoral heads thus compromising psoas function. These concepts will be elaborated upon throughout the book.

For demonstration of these concepts, visit www.IIHFE.com/the-psoas-solution.

To better appreciate the functional role of the psoas in stabilizing and/or moving the hip, spine, and pelvis (which will also be examined throughout the various exercise patterns), a review of joint centration and open- and closed-chain motion is warranted.

Joint Centration

Joint centration, a term that will be used throughout this book, refers to the ability to align and control one's joint, whether in a static posture (non-moving) or in a dynamic position (see image below). Centration is achieved by the coordinated effort of the nervous system receiving feedback from the proprioceptive system and executing the most advantageous motor strategy to control the joint(s) required for the task in hand.

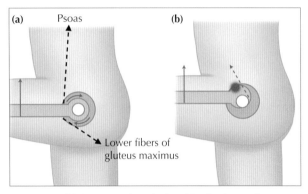

(a) Optimal hip centration during hip flexion—the psoas and lower gluteal fibers work with the other deep hip muscles to maintain the femoral head within the acetabulum during movement of the leg. (b) Non-optimal hip centration during hip flexion—the femoral head shifts anteriorly and superiorly within the acetabulum when the psoas and other deep stabilizers are unable to optimally control the joint position.

Joint centration implies a joint position in which the cartilaginous surfaces are in maximum contact and the forces acting upon the joint are appropriately distributed across the joint surfaces (Kolar et al. 2013). Centration enables the optimal positioning and control of one's joints so that there is a greater ability to:

- activate all the muscles around the joint when required for postural control and movement;
- provide the appropriate proprioceptive feedback from the joint and soft tissue receptors;
- prevent excessive joint compression (resulting from too much myofascial activation), uncontrolled joint motion (hypermobility), and/or overstretching or strain of the joint's soft tissue structures (joint capsule, ligaments, muscles, and fascia).

A requirement for optimal centration is that there is coordinated activity in each of the muscles acting upon a joint. This enables simultaneous centration as well as a well-controlled *axis of rotation*—the ideal, theoretical point around which a joint moves. Too much muscle activity in all the muscles surrounding a joint leads to over-compression. Imbalances where there is too much activity of one or more muscles relative to their *functional synergists* (muscles that work together to stabilize or move a joint) disrupts centration, and therefore affects optimal centration and motion.

When there is balanced muscle activity between the deep and superficial muscles, the femoral head remains relatively centered within the acetabulum, regardless of the range of motion. When compromised—for example by over-activating the superficial gluteus maximus, hamstrings, and/or hip rotators relative to the deep fibers and psoas—the femoral head loses its ideal position of centration and translates anteriorly. This then overstretches the anterior joint capsule and compromises soft tissue structures, such as the labrum. This is a common scenario in the cascade of events that ultimately leads to femoroacetabular impingement syndrome (FAI), labral tears, and other degenerative changes of the hip.

Similarly, when the psoas, along with the other muscles of the deep myofascial system (DMS), balances out the activity of the superficial erectors and abdominals, the spine remains well centered. However, with inhibition of the psoas, transversus abdominis, or multifidi, and compensatory overactivity of the superficial muscles, spinal centration is compromised. As discussed above in the case of the hip, this prolonged non-optimal strategy ultimately contributes to degenerative disc and joint disease of the spine. These concepts will be expanded upon throughout the book.

Joint centration is a dynamic process and is therefore affected by many factors. Factors that can *de-centrate* or contribute to non-optimal joint alignment and control include:

- Neural inhibition secondary to spinal nerve root irritation.
  - Disc pathology (bulges or herniation) affecting any of the thoracic or lumbar nerves can impact corresponding muscle function around the trunk, spine, and/or hips, which in turn leads to compensation and muscle imbalances.
- Muscle imbalances secondary to trauma, surgery, or inflammation.
  - Trauma, surgery, or joint inflammation can contribute to muscle inhibition, primarily of the deeper or intrinsic joint muscles, which can ultimately result in loss of motor control.
  - Inhibition leads to compensatory overuse in certain muscles—generally the superficial muscles—which further compromises optimal centration.
- Improper training.
  - Improper exercise patterning (e.g. squatting too deeply for one's range of motion and moving into excessive posterior tilt and lumbar spine flexion) and improper cuing (e.g. over-activating or squeezing the glutes at the top of the squatting pattern) can contribute to over-activation of certain muscles relative to others, thus affecting joint alignment and control.

An individual's success in performing at an optimal level, relieving chronic tightness or discomfort, and minimizing the risk of injury is ultimately impacted by their ability to achieve joint centration. The goal during any rehabilitation and/or training program is to choose the most appropriate exercise patterns, cues, and strategies that improve and/or maintain ideal joint centration. This topic will be central to developing the exercise patterns that will be discussed in future chapters.

Clinical Consideration

Joint centration is often considered an esoteric concept, therefore its use as a valid assessment tool often comes under criticism. Most of the misunderstanding stems from the inability of practitioners to accurately determine whether or not a joint is properly centrated. Because few individuals are actually trained in its evaluation, joint centration is either discarded as an invalid assessment tool, or given the perfunctory glance test ("I think it is doing/not doing what I think it should" or "It looks like it is/is not moving the way it should").

While one can observe what is happening in a particular region of the body, it is impossible to accurately determine what is actually happening at the joint level on the basis of visual inspection alone. Palpation is the most accurate and reliable method for evaluating joint position and movement.

Like any clinical ability, palpating for joint centration is a skill, honed only by placing one's hands on and evaluating many joints—both those that are well aligned and controlled and those that are not so well aligned and controlled.

A thorough understanding of structural anatomy, biomechanics (where a joint is ideally positioned and how it should optimally move), and motor control (how the neuromyofascial system is affecting the joint position during a particular posture or movement) is a prerequisite for being able to determine whether or not a joint is ideally centrated.

While not every individual will need that specific level of evaluation, the clinician or fitness professional may have clients or patients that present with chronic low back or hip issues that could be related to non-optimal joint centration. Because they are presenting for treatment, most individuals that are presenting with chronic tightness, pain, and/or loss of performance should be evaluated for joint centration and more importantly their control strategy. If one's profession does not allow hands-on palpation, it can be beneficial to establish a working relationship with a practitioner who is trained to evaluate for joint centration. In lieu of putting one's hands the individual, decision-making must then rely solely on the information provided by one's eyes, assessment, and experience.

Open- and Closed-Chain Motion

The terms "open chain" and "closed chain" are often mentioned when discussing movement of the lower kinetic chain. The *kinetic chain* refers to the structural and neural connections between adjoining segments of the body. A movement is considered to be *open chain* when the distal aspect of the kinetic chain—the foot or other segment of the lower extremity in the example of the lower extremity—is not in contact with a surface and is therefore not generally considered to influence proximal joint motion (see "Clinical Consideration" opposite for more on this discussion). When the distal aspect of the kinetic chain is in contact with a surface, so that it influences motion at the more proximal joints, the movement is considered to be *closed chain*.

An example of open-chain motion of the hip is a standing hip flexion pattern, in which the hip is flexing, but movement of the lower extremity is not affecting the position of the hip. Conversely, when squatting, the foot is in contact with the ground and therefore, through its impact upon the tibia and femur, motion at the hip joint is influenced.

Open chain hip flexion of the right hip (near right image); closed chain hip flexion during a squat (far right image).

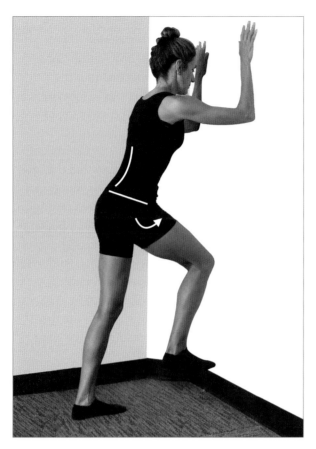
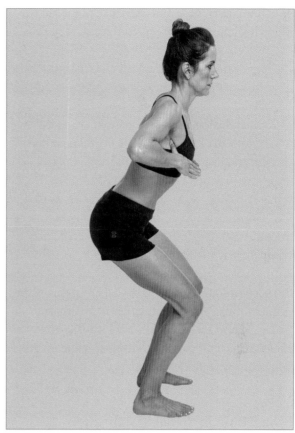

Clinical Consideration

Open-chain movements are thought to be isolated joint motions that do not necessarily have the ability to affect distal areas of the body. For example, the ankle and foot are generally not regarded as having an ability to influence motion of the hip when the foot is off the ground, such as when sitting or lying. However, the ankle and foot complex is neurologically linked to the entire kinetic chain. Clinically, changes in hip motion and strength have been observed after centrating—centrating the ankle and foot, even when performed in a seated or supine position with the foot not in contact with any surface. This is largely why such a strong emphasis is placed upon centrating as many joints as possible during rehabilitation or training, regardless of the position of the body.

Functional Anatomy of the Psoas

This section will look at the PMj and PMn as the two component parts of the psoas complex. Since the PMj will send fibers into the superior ramus of the pubis in the absence of the PMn (Stecco 2015, Myers 2014), this section will identify the combined actions of these muscles. From this point on, the psoas major and minor will collectively be referred to simply as the *psoas*.

Because of the psoas' location deep in the abdominal cavity, actual in vivo (in a living body) studies of this muscle are limited. Most commonly accepted actions of the psoas have been derived from cadaveric studies, which consequently limit its actions to what occurs when the distal end of the muscle (insertion) is brought closer to the proximal end of the muscle (origin), or vice versa.

Therefore, most texts and literature point out the following commonly accepted roles of the psoas:

- Hip flexion and external rotation in open chain or when the femur moves around the fixed pelvis
- Spinal flexion in closed chain or when the legs are fixed and the pelvis moves around the femoral heads

It has also been suggested that the psoas, as part of the "iliopsoas complex," is the only muscle that has the potential to flex the hip toward the end range of hip flexion (Sahrmann 2002).

It has commonly been taught that the psoas is the primary muscle that contributes to an anterior pelvic tilt and increased lumbar lordosis. The psoas' impact on pelvic and lumbar spine posture will be investigated below.

Psoas' Role in Spinal Stabilization

The broad and intricate attachments of the psoas suggest that it has a much more involved and dynamic role in function than previously noted. The various attachments at every vertebral level from the lower thoracic and lumbar spine, and the intricate fascial attachments into various muscles around the spine and pelvis, provide evidence that the psoas is much more than a flexor of the hip and the spine. This elaborate design suggests that the psoas probably has a more significant role in stability of the spine and pelvis, as well as of the hip, than has been previously attributed to it.

The psoas is considered a powerful axial compressor—and therefore stabilizer—of the lumbar spine (Bogduk 2005). Because of its proximity to the spine, the psoas has not been shown to contribute significantly to spinal movement, such as lateral bending and rotation (Bogduk 2005). Therefore, it is more likely that the psoas functions as a stabilizer of the spine during these movements.

Further evidence of the psoas' contribution to spinal stability has been demonstrated in the research. Electromyography (EMG), utilizing fine wire needle electrodes inserted into the psoas bilaterally during a lying single-leg raise, demonstrated activity in both the leg being raised and in the psoas on the opposite side to the leg that was being lifted (Hu et al. 2011). Consistent with these findings, it has been suggested that the psoas aids in lumbar spine stability to counteract the anterior shear forces that are created during hip flexion (Gibbons 2007, McGill 2007). Bilateral psoas activation provides frontal plane stability of the spine (Hu et al. 2011, Penning 2002, Andersson et al. 1995) and limits excessive side bending and rotation while lifting (Sullivan 1989). It has been proposed that the psoas supports the trunk on the pelvis and prevents buckling of the spine (Penning 2000).

Contracting eccentrically, the psoas aids in the control of contralateral side bending (Gibbons 2007). Additionally, the psoas will eccentrically lengthen, acting as a stabilizer of the lumbar spine and controlling the amount of spinal extension during overhead motion or backward bending (Osar 2015). This prevents over-compression of the lumbar facet joints and overstretching of the anterior spinal ligaments as the spine is extended.

Although it has been thought that the psoas has a role in spinal flexion, when the pelvis is fixed the psoas pulls the lumbar spine into more lordosis (Penning 2002). In a standing position, the psoas may contribute to forward bending; however, it is more likely that the muscle is shortening as a result of the abdominals and gravity simultaneously flexing the lumbar spine from this position. The psoas may contribute to forward bending and flexion of the spine in the upright position if these actions are being performed against a resistance. During a Roll-up (image near left) (see Chapter 6) or sit-up the psoas may play a more active role in spinal flexion and decreasing lumbar lordosis than in standing. With the trunk fixed as in an Articulating Bridge

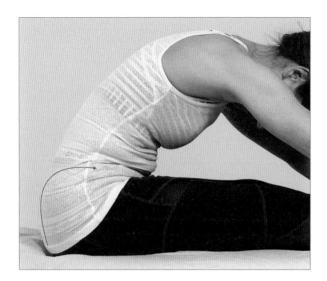

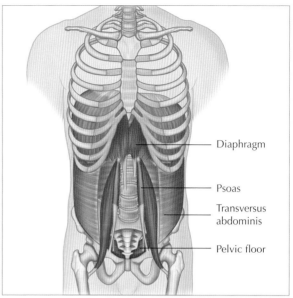

— Diaphragm

— Psoas

— Transversus abdominis

— Pelvic floor

pattern (also referred to as a *Pelvic Tilt* pattern—see Chapter 2) or in a reverse crunch exercise, it is likely that certain portions of the psoas assist in posterior rotation of the pelvis and in segmental flexion of the lumbar spine, which decrease or lessen the lumbar lordosis.

Psoas' Impact Upon the Pelvis

Traditionally, the psoas has been thought to contribute to increasing anterior rotation (tilt) of the pelvis. However, recall that the only attachments of the psoas directly to the pelvis lie anteriorly on the superior pubic ramus and into the pelvic floor. These attachments suggest that the psoas will posteriorly rotate the pelvis rather than anteriorly rotate it (Gibbons 2007, Osar 2015).

Even though the psoas directly attaches across the anterior surface of the sacroiliac joints, no direct link of the psoas to these joints has been studied so far. It has been suggested that the psoas creates a stabilizing force across the sacroiliac joint (Gibbons 2007). Research has demonstrated that muscles having either direct or fascial connections to the sacroiliac joint—multifidus, gluteus maximus, and biceps femoris for

Note the psoas' attachments to both the anterior pelvis and pelvic floor (image above). These attachments suggest that the pelvis contributes to posterior pelvic rotation and assists in controlling anterior pelvic rotation.

example—contribute to stabilization of this joint (Lee 2012, Richardson et al. 2004, Vleeming 2012). The psoas most likely plays a significant role in the stabilization of the sacroiliac joint; however, more research in that area is required at this time.

Psoas' Relationship to the Lumbar Multifidus

In respect of spinal stabilization, the muscle that is the most analogous to the psoas is the multifidus. It is located on the posterior aspect of the lumbar spine, and is the most medial and deepest of the lumbar muscles. The deeper fibers of the multifidus arise from the posterior aspect of the spine and insert two levels below their origin. The superficial fibers arise from the spinous processes and extend three levels below their origin. The fibers of the lower lumbar division of the multifidus insert into the pelvis, sacrum, and sacroiliac joint.

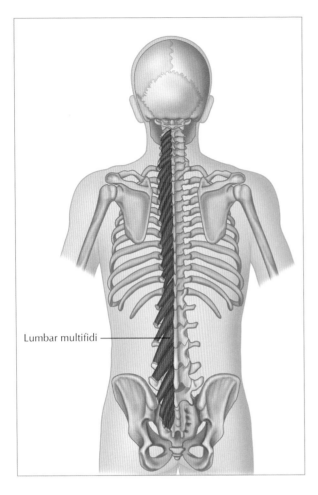

Lumbar multifidi

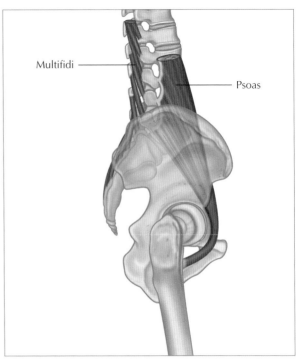

Multifidi

Psoas

The deeper fibers of the multifidus demonstrate a low level of activity, even at rest (tonic activity), and thus are more involved in segmental vertebral control and postural stability (Richardson et al. 2004). These deeper fibers demonstrate anticipatory reactions on EMG results, which means that they contract prior to actual movement, demonstrating that they have similar characteristics to other deep muscles, such as the transversus abdominis and the pelvic floor muscles (Richardson et al. 2004). The superficial fibers tend to have a greater extensor torque, or an ability to extend the lumbar spine. Collectively, both divisions of the multifidus work synergistically with the psoas to stabilize the lumbar spine and the sacroiliac joints, thus preventing excessive shear and translation forces (image above right).

Similarly, both the multifidus and psoas demonstrate a decrease in cross-sectional size (atrophy) in individuals with low back pain and/ or unilateral sciatica (Barker et al. 2004, Dangaria and Naesh 1998). Specific exercises targeted at the multifidus and psoas have been shown to be effective in improving the size of these muscles as well as in decreasing pain in patients with degenerative disc disease (Seongho et al. 2014). Exercise and educational strategies that enhance the activation of the DMS have been shown to clinically improve both psoas and multifidus function and thereby enhance spinal stability (Osar 2015). Strategies for improving co-activation of the psoas and multifidus will be presented in Chapter 3.

Psoas' Role in Hip Function

The psoas has traditionally been thought of as the body's primary hip flexor. Recent evidence suggests that as the psoas contracts, it creates axial compression of both the spine and the femoral head (Gibbons 2005ab, 2007); thus, the psoas *centrates* (aligns and controls) the femoral head within the acetabulum.

As the hip is brought into flexion by the primary hip flexors—the rectus femoris, tensor fasciae latae, and sartorius—the psoas aids this movement by compressing and maintaining the position of the femoral head within the acetabulum. It therefore aids hip flexion by maintaining the axis of rotation, rather than working as a prime mover. While the psoas may assist external rotation, it is more likely that it functions as a stabilizer of the femoral head within the acetabulum during the movement, rather than actually contributing to the movement.

Psoas' Relationship to the Iliacus

The iliacus (image right) deserves mention, since many texts refer to the iliacus and psoas collectively as the *iliopsoas* because of their similar tendon attachment into the lesser trochanter of the femur. The iliacus originates from within the pelvis (iliac fossa) and proceeds over the iliopubic eminence of the pelvis, before inserting into the lesser trochanter of the femur. While the psoas and iliacus share a similar attachment point on the femur, each has its own individual tendinous attachment (McGill 2007) and separate nerve innervations (Retchford et al. 2013) indicating they function independent of each other.

Because of its shorter lever arm and proximity to the hip joint, contrary to the psoas the iliacus likely has a strong ability to flex the hip. In fact, it has been suggested that the psoas has a negligible role in hip flexion, and that the rectus femoris, tensor fasciae latae, and sartorius are more efficient hip flexors than both the psoas and iliacus (Gibbons 2007). Collectively, it has been suggested that the psoas and iliacus may play a role in hip stabilization similar to the rotator cuff muscles at the shoulder (Lewis et al. 2007).

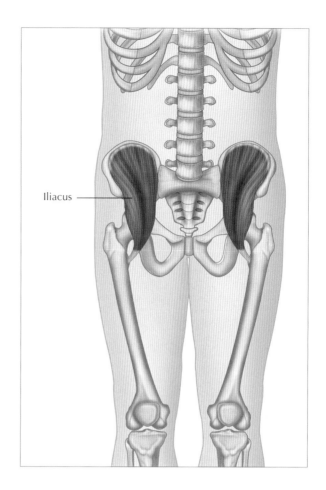

Iliacus

The iliacus has been shown to play a role in stabilizing the hip in the late phase of gait (Retchfort et al. 2013). When the femur is fixed, the iliacus is a primary contributor in anteriorly rotating (tilting) the pelvis. By increasing anterior rotation of the pelvis, the iliacus can indirectly contribute to increasing the lordotic curve of the lumbar spine.

The psoas and iliacus likely act as *functional antagonists* (two muscles that theoretically oppose each other, but collectively function together):

- The two muscles collectively contribute to hip flexion—the psoas centrates the femoral head, while the iliacus flexes the hip.
- The iliacus anteriorly tilts the pelvis, which increases lumbar lordosis, while the psoas posteriorly tilts the pelvis and compresses the lumbar spine, thereby counteracting the action of the iliacus.

This synergistic relationship provides both spine stability and control of hip movement that is required for performing functional activities, while at the same time decreasing the risk of sustaining overuse injuries of the joints or soft tissue structures.

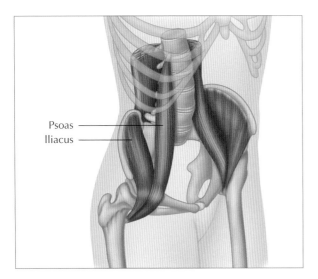

Psoas' Relationship to the Gluteus Maximus

The psoas and gluteus maximus have traditionally been considered antagonists: the gluteus maximus extending the hip, and the psoas flexing it. Similarly, it has been thought that the psoas pulls the pelvis into anterior rotation (commonly referred to as *anterior pelvic tilt*) and the gluteus maximus pulls it into posterior rotation (or *posterior pelvic tilt*). Recent evidence, however, suggests that these muscles have a relationship that is synergistic rather than antagonistic.

The gluteus maximus attaches proximally to the lateral aspect of the iliac crest and sacrum; these attachments are continuous with the posterior fascia covering both the sacrum and the multifidus. The gluteal fascia also adjoins to the thoracolumbar fascia, thereby functionally connecting the gluteus maximus

with the contralateral latissimus dorsi. This myofascial connection is referred to by several names, including the *posterior oblique chain* (Osar 2012), *posterior oblique sling* (Lee 2012), or *back functional line* (Myers 2014) (see image below).

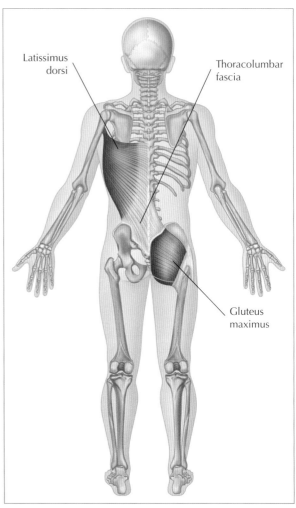

The superficial fibers of the gluteus maximus attach to the iliotibial band and the gluteal tuberosity (posterior aspect of the femur), while the deeper gluteal fibers attach only to the gluteal tuberosity. The deeper, inferior fibers of the gluteus maximus arise from the lower sacrum and coccyx; these fibers cross the sacroiliac joint and attach just lateral to the posterior superior iliac spine, and fascially blend with the sacrotuberous ligament and fascia of the deep intrinsic hip muscles.

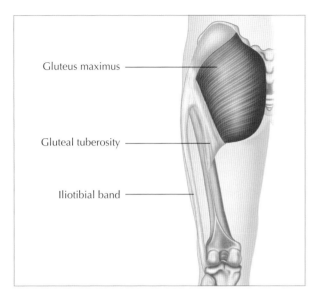

Gluteus maximus

Gluteal tuberosity

Iliotibial band

Just after midstance (image below), the psoas eccentrically lengthens to control the femoral head within the acetabulum, and decelerates the rate and amount of both hip and spine extension.

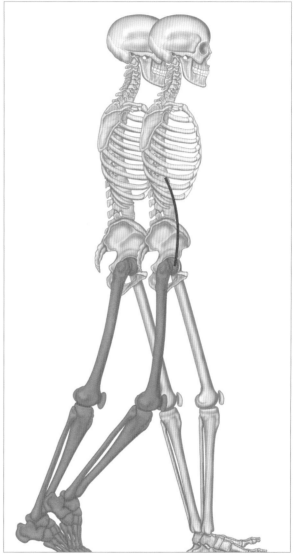

While the superficial fibers of the gluteus maximus have the primary role of hip extension and pelvic stabilization, the deeper, lower fibers of this muscle draw the femoral head posteriorly within the acetabulum (Gibbons 2005ab, Gibbons 2007). The deeper fibers of the gluteus maximus are functional synergists with the psoas in the centration of the femoral head within the acetabulum during movement of the hip. Ideal co-activation of these two muscles provides the optimal compression required to stabilize the femoral head during hip movement and hence lower extremity movement.

Training to improve synergy between the psoas and the gluteus maximus is vital in improving hip function and preventing hip impingement syndromes. Exercise strategies for training this synergy will be included in later chapters.

Psoas' Role in Gait

Since it is the only muscle that directly connects the spine with the lower extremity, the psoas is key during the gait cycle. The psoas—along with the iliacus—demonstrates peak EMG activity during two distinct phases of the gait cycle: terminal stance and the early swing phase (Michaud 2011). During hip flexion, the psoas assists the iliacus in flexion of the advancing leg.

It is likely that the contralateral psoas is stabilizing the spine during hip extension; however, more information is required to substantiate this theory. It is important to recognize that, although the psoas does not demonstrate EMG activity through the rest of the gait cycle, this does not suggest that it is not active in its role of spinal and hip stabilization. Future research may bring to light how the psoas is functioning through the entire gait cycle.

Improving the psoas' ability to centrate the hip (the femoral head within the acetabulum) plays an important role in improving an individual's gait. Exercises to improve the muscle's contribution to hip flexion and controlling hip extension will be included in later chapters.

Psoas' Role in Respiration

Given its intimate fascial connections to the diaphragm, transversus abdominis, and quadratus lumborum at the thoracolumbar junction (TLJ) and the pelvic floor inferiorly, the psoas likely functions as an important stabilizer of the spine during respiration (Gibbons 2007, Osar 2015). The role of the psoas in optimal breathing will be expanded on in Chapter 2.

Below is an image of the psoas and its fascial connections to the diaphragm, transversus abdominis, and pelvic floor. The intimate relationship between these structures suggests that the psoas has a dual role in supporting both respiration and stabilization.

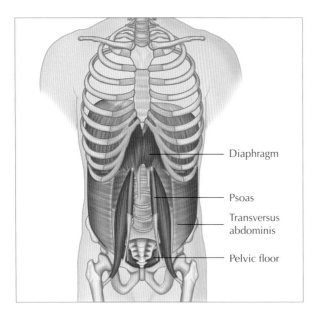

Diaphragm

Psoas

Transversus abdominis

Pelvic floor

Psoas' Role in Upper Body Movement

Although the psoas has a direct connection to the lower extremities, it does not have a similar relationship with the upper extremities; however, its function during upper body movement patterns is no less important. As discussed earlier, the psoas will stabilize the spine, pelvis, and hips, thereby creating a more solid anchor for expressing upper body strength. Additionally, the psoas stabilizes the spine, thus protecting it from over-compression or excessive/uncontrolled shear-type forces that could potentially cause injury when lifting, pushing, pulling, and/or throwing.

Summary of Psoas Functions

Psoas functions at the trunk, spine, and pelvis
- Stabilizes the TLJ, lumbar spine, and pelvis.
- Contributes to spinal flexion when either the legs or the trunk are fixed.
- Assists posterior pelvic rotation.
- Eccentrically controls spinal extension when bending backwards and spinal flexion during a deep-squatting or forward bending pattern (at the point where the lumbar spine begins to flex).

Psoas functions at the hip
- Centrates the femoral head within the acetabulum.
- Assists hip flexion by stabilizing the femoral head within the acetabulum.
- Eccentrically controls hip extension.

Summary: Functional Anatomy

To provide a more complete perspective of the psoas, this chapter has highlighted the functional anatomy of the muscle, including its attachments and multiple functions in relation to the trunk, spine, pelvis, and hips. The incredible communication that the psoas has with a variety of myofascial structures within the thoracic and lumbar spine, as well as within the pelvic and hip complexes, has been identified. Movements relating to the hips, spine, and pelvis have been defined in order to help establish common terminology that will be discussed in later chapters. To develop a more efficient postural and movement strategy, the incorporation and training of the psoas' multiple functions involving the trunk, spine, pelvis, and hips will be the focus of subsequent chapters.

1. The psoas has extensive fascial attachments to the trunk, spine, pelvis, and hips. Additionally, it fascially attaches to several muscles within these regions, including the diaphragm, quadratus lumborum, transversus abdominis, pelvic floor, and iliacus.
2. Emerging evidence suggests that the psoas' primary role is stabilization of the spine, pelvis, and hips to allow smooth and coordinated movement, without creating excessive strain upon the joints or soft tissue structures in these regions.
3. The psoas performs a function of stabilizing the spine and pelvis during a variety of movements. The muscle axially compresses (stiffens) the spine to stabilize it against anterior shear forces that are created by the lifting of the leg during hip flexion. When contracting isometrically, the psoas will maintain the lumbar lordosis. It contributes to increasing the lumbar lordosis when the TPC is not aligned and stable.
4. Trunk and spine flexion: the psoas assists trunk flexion and posterior rotation of the pelvis in certain movements and exercises.

Generally it aids flexion of the trunk when the pelvis and hips are anchored, as in a sit-up movement. The muscle will assist posterior rotation of the pelvis and segmentally flex the spine (reducing the lordotic curve in the lumbar spine) when the trunk is the fixed point and the legs are being lifted. It will counteract anterior rotation of the pelvis created by the hip flexors.

5. Spinal rotation: the psoas stabilizes the spine and pelvis by maintaining an aligned (stacked) position, so that rotation of the trunk and spine occurs around a vertical or longitudinal axis. This prevents excessive lateral shear forces from occurring through the spine during rotation.
6. Spinal extension and lateral flexion: the psoas eccentrically lengthens to control extension and side bending of the spine. This serves to protect these regions against excessive extension-type movements that could potentially over-compress spinal joints or stress soft tissue structures.
7. Hip flexion and extension: the psoas assists hip flexion by stabilizing the femoral head in the acetabulum. It maintains the position of the femoral head in the acetabulum as the other primary hip flexors—iliacus and rectus femoris—flex the hip. The psoas functions synergistically with the gluteus maximus to stabilize the femoral head in the acetabulum during hip movement. The muscle has a negligible role in hip rotation, other than stabilizing the joint during movement. The psoas controls hip extension during activities such as walking, running, and lunging. It will eccentrically lengthen to protect the hip against excessive extension-type movements, thus preventing excessive anterior translation of the femoral head within the acetabulum.
8. Respiration: the psoas assists breathing by stabilizing the trunk and spine. It functions

as a stabilizer of the TLJ of the spine, thus providing an anchor for optimal function of the diaphragm.

9. Pushing and pulling: the psoas functions as a stabilizer of the spine, pelvis, and hips while lifting, pushing, and/or pulling with the upper extremities.

10. Gait: as the only muscle directly connecting the spine to the hip, the psoas has multiple roles during gait. It stabilizes the trunk, spine, and pelvis, assists hip flexion of the advancing leg, and eccentrically controls hip extension from the mid-stance through the terminal-stance phase of the gait cycle.

Three-dimensional Breathing

A s mentioned in the previous chapter, the psoas has a significant role in breathing. While it does not directly influence the respiratory process, it does play a major part in the stabilization of the trunk and spine during the respiratory cycle. This chapter will briefly describe the respiratory process, introduce the role of the psoas in three-dimensional breathing, and develop a paradigm for integrating psoas function into three-dimensional breathing.

Anatomy of Three-dimensional Breathing

The question often arises as to what the importance of breathing is when everyone seems to be doing an adequate job of it—after all, they are alive and therefore evidently taking in enough oxygen and not passing out because of a lack of it. While on the surface it may appear that everyone is alive and well, the signs of non-optimal respiratory strategies subtly reveal themselves in a host of conditions, including (but not limited to) fatigue, sensitivity to touch, chronic tightness, chronic low back and/ or shoulder discomfort, muscle cramps, muscle weakness, anxiety, and high blood pressure.

A critical review of individuals who failed low back surgery reported that dysfunction of the diaphragm may contribute to continued issues in these patients (Bordoni and Marelli 2016). Therefore it is likely that respiration is too frequently overlooked as a contributing factor to both overall health and musculoskeletal dysfunction, and consequently warrants a closer look.

Three-dimensional breathing refers to the ability to expand and relax the thoracic, abdominal, and pelvic cavities superior to inferior (top to bottom),

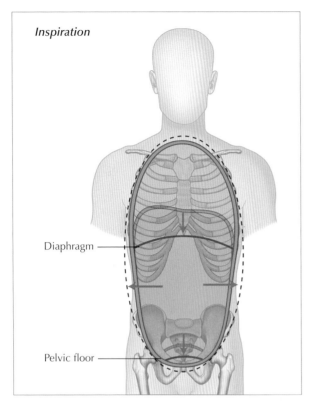
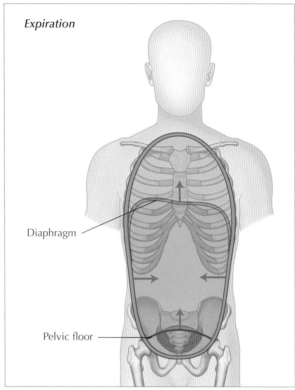
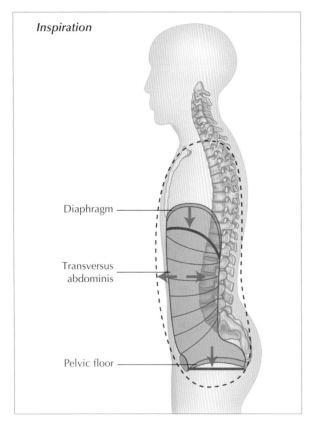
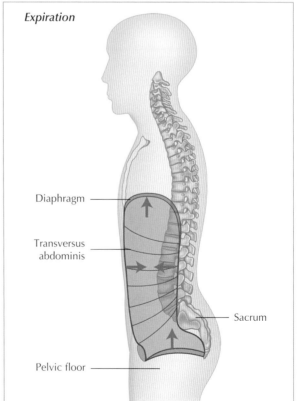

Three-dimensional breathing—front and side views of inspiration (left) and expiration (right); note how the diaphragm and pelvic floor move synchronously within the TPC during each phase of the breath cycle.

laterally (side to side), and anteroposteriorly (front to back). Three-dimensional movement involves increasing during inhalation and decreasing during exhalation the volumes of all three cavities (images on p. 40).

The goal of breath retraining is to improve the capacity to use all regions of the thoracopelvic cylinder (TPC) during the respiratory cycle. There are times when one region will predominate over another; therefore the individual must be able to access all three—thoracic, abdominal, and pelvic—to ensure that these are available when needed.

Functions of Three-dimensional Breathing

Although oxygenation of the body is the most commonly identified goal of respiration, there are in fact five primary functions of optimal three-dimensional breathing.

1. *Oxygenation.* The overall goal of optimal breathing is to oxygenate the body and to expel carbon dioxide to sustain life. Three-dimensional breathing is the optimal way to accomplish this goal, without the need for compensatory strategies to fulfill these requirements for living. Because there is generally better oxygen perfusion with each breath, three-dimensional breathing requires fewer breaths per minute, which can in turn theoretically lower one's resting heart rate and blood pressure.

2. *Stability and mobility.* Three-dimensional breathing is the most efficient way to use the diaphragm and other muscles of the trunk, spine, and pelvis to regulate the pressures between the three cavities. With optimal control of internal pressures, the trunk, spine, and pelvis are stabilized at the same time as the respiratory demands are being met. Additionally, this breathing strategy

facilitates activation of the psoas and other muscles that are fascially and neurologically connected with the diaphragm; this provides the requisite stabilization for the TPC and hips without the need to compensate by overusing the myofascial system. Throughout this book, three-dimensional breathing will be discussed as a means of developing and maintaining TPC stability as well as of increasing the activity of the psoas and other muscles of the deep myofascial system (DMS).

Additionally, any movement of the diaphragm causes a pulling action on its attachments, which acts to rhythmically mobilize the spine and rib cage. Thoracic mobility—and thus stability—is compromised when the psoas does not adequately stabilize the thoracolumbar junction (TLJ) and the diaphragm remains in an elevated and flattened position resulting in insufficient inferior and/or posterior movement of the diaphragm (Bordoni and Marelli 2016). Over time, non-optimal breathing leads to thoracic rigidity, which in turn compromises optimal three-dimensional expansion of the rib cage (Osar 2015). Overusing the myofascial system for trunk, spine, pelvis and/or hip stability is a common compensation for non-optimal pressure regulation within the cavities. Over-relying on muscle force as a compensatory strategy for core stabilization will consequently also contribute to diminished thoracic mobility. This concept will be expanded on in the section "Common Breathing Dysfunctions" near the end of this chapter.

3. *Organ health and digestion.* While the role of breathing is rarely related to organ health, the *motility* of an organ (its natural, inherent ebb and flow) and its *mobility* (its ability to freely move within its specific space) are related to movement of the diaphragm. When optimal three-dimensional breathing takes place, the contraction of the diaphragm causes it to move inferiorly and push the internal organs down toward the pelvis during inspiration. The reflexive contraction of the pelvic floor

and the elastic recoil of the trunk, lungs, and abdominal wall compress the abdominal organs and push them back up to their resting position upon expiration. Three-dimensional breathing thus plays an important role in improving motility of the gastrointestinal system (Massery 2006, Chapter 39:695–717), as well as in maintaining mobility of the organs and internal fascial network.

Additionally, the diaphragm helps support the lower esophageal sphincter thereby preventing the flow of stomach acid back into the esophagus (image below). Gastroesophageal reflux disease (GERD), commonly referred to as heartburn, indigestion, or acid stomach, is a common condition in asthmatics as well as in many individuals who present with thoracic rigidity and loss of balance between the psoas, diaphragm, and inner muscles compared with the more superficial abdominal muscles and erector spinae. Clinically, GERD is prevalent in a significant number of patients who have an inspiratory (elevated) position of the diaphragm and hyperextension at the TLJ. Specific retraining aimed at restoring more optimal diaphragmatic breathing has been shown to improve GERD symptoms (Casale et al. 2016).

4. *Circulation.* Similarly, any movement of the diaphragm physically aids vascular and lymph flow through the abdominal, thoracic, and pelvic regions, thus supporting optimal organ health. As mentioned in point 1 above, three-dimensional breathing also allows more optimal exchange of gases, thereby decreasing the overall cardiovascular demands on the system. Increased heart rate and blood pressure are common signs of an inadequate gas exchange that may be related to a non-optimal breathing strategy.

5. *Relaxation.* One of the greatest benefits of three-dimensional breathing is that it improves parasympathetic nervous system activity while reducing sympathetic nervous system activity (Umphred 2007). When the body is in a parasympathetic state, the nervous system can focus on the tasks required to support repair, regeneration, and vitality, thus decreasing muscle damage and preventing overall inflammation. Common signs of *sympathetic dominance* or overactivity of the sympathetic nervous system include an elevated resting heart rate, elevated blood pressure, rapid and shallow breathing, muscle fatigue and achiness, joint discomfort, and general anxiety.

It is important to note that the ability to perform these five functions is reliant upon the competence of the psoas, intercostals, abdominals, spinal erector spinae, and pelvic floor muscles to provide a stable base, so that the diaphragm can ideally function as a piston within the TPC.

The diaphragm as a piston within the TPC—During inspiration, the diaphragm contracts and lowers (image p. 43). This action pushes the abdominals contents down and thereby stretches both the abdominal wall and the pelvic floor thereby increasing the volume of the abdominal and pelvic cavities.

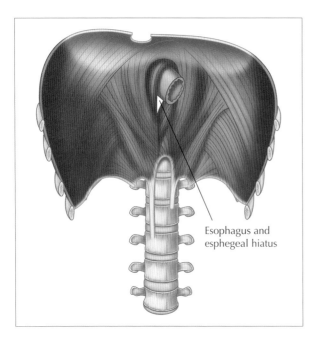

Esophagus and esphegeal hiatus

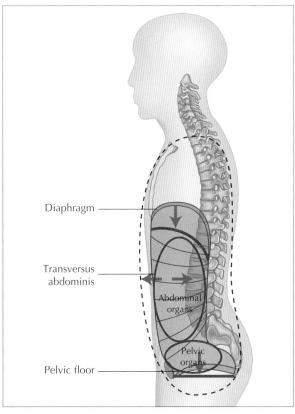

As the diaphragm contracts it pushes the abdominal and pelvic contents down into the pelvic cavity and thereby activates the pelvic floor.

Muscles Most Responsible for Quiet Respiration		
	Primary	**Accessory**
Inspiration	Diaphragm Intercostals Levatores costarum Scalenes	Sternocleidomastoid Serratus posterior superior Iliocostalis thoracis Subclavius Pectoralis minor
Expiration	Elastic recoil of the lungs, diaphragm, pelvic floor, joints of the thoracic cage, muscles and fascia surrounding the thoracic cage	Transversus thoracis Subcostales Iliocostalis lumborum Quadratus lumborum Serratus posterior inferior

The biomechanics associated with three-dimensional breathing will be discussed in a later section.

Muscles of Respiration

While it is generally agreed that the diaphragm is the primary muscle of respiration, many other muscles are required to assist *quiet respiration* (how one breathes at rest). For example, the intercostals, levatores costarum, and scalenes each play a significant role in expanding the vertical and transverse dimensions of the thorax. Quiet expiration occurs primarily as a result of the elastic recoil that has been stored up in the lungs, diaphragm, pelvic floor, and joints of the thoracic cage itself, as well as in the vast network of muscles and fascia surrounding the thoracic cage. During rapid or forced inhalation, such as occurs while exercising, the accessory muscles play a more significant role in supporting the respiratory process.

Psoas' Role in Breathing

As discussed in Chapter 1, proximally the psoas attaches at the TLJ and fascially connects with the spinal attachments of the diaphragm; distally, it fascially blends with the pelvic floor. The pelvic floor is the bottom of the TPC and eccentrically contracts during inspiration to resist the increasing abdominal pressure and inferior movement of the abdominal and pelvic organs. In essence, the diaphragm and pelvic floor are synchronous structures and move within the TPC during breathing; they move inferiorly during inspiration and superiorly during expiration, creating a piston-type effect within the TPC (Bordoni and Zanier 2013). For visualization of these motions, visit the informed health website at https://www.informedhealth.org/pelvic-floor-training.2288.en.html.

The psoas is the functional link between the diaphragm and pelvic floor, acting as a stabilizer of

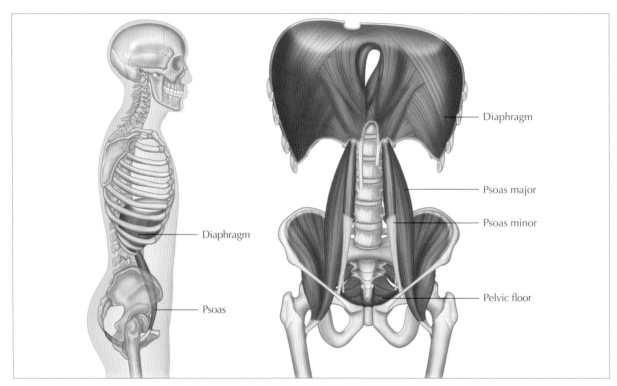

The psoas is myofascially linked to the diaphragm and pelvic floor; this relationship provides spinal stability during respiration.

the lower thoracic and lumbar spine as well as of the pelvis (images above).

In this manner the psoas provides a force to maintain the stability of the TPC during respiration and movements that alter an individual's breathing strategy. This construct enables the body to meet its respiratory and stabilization requirements through a myriad of situations that would otherwise challenge breathing or postural control.

In turn, three-dimensional breathing helps activate the muscles that are fascially and functionally linked with the diaphragm, including (but not limited to) the psoas, transversus abdominis, quadratus lumborum, and pelvic floor. Research has demonstrated a co-activation of the transversus abdominis and pelvic floor prior to movement (Richardson et al. 2004, Hodges et al. 2013). Research into spinal stabilization has demonstrated a similar response to other deep spinal stabilizers including the multifidus (Richardson et al. 2004, Hodges et al. 2013). Since this *feedforward*

activation strategy is demonstrated in several muscles directly attaching to the spine and pelvis, it is likely that the psoas shares a similar response and activates just prior to movement (Osar 2015). Pre-activation of the psoas prior to movement would theoretically provide segmental stabilization of the TPC against the pull of the diaphragm. Three-dimensional breathing in combination with specific mental imagery or visual cues can be instrumental in improving timing and control of the DMS (Osar 2015). Specific training to improve activation of the DMS will be discussed in Chapter 3.

Biomechanics of Three-dimensional Breathing

A *respiratory cycle* is defined as taking a breath in (an inspiration) followed by a corresponding breath out (an expiration). Under ideal circumstances, this process should be coordinated and relatively effortless. During the majority of life activities, respiration is under autonomic control, meaning that it does not have to be consciously thought about; however, an individual can consciously alter their breathing pattern when speaking or singing, or during activities such as meditation and exercise.

During *quiet respiration*, the respiratory strategy performed under rest and non-stressful situations, the Cleveland Clinic suggests 12 to 20 breaths per minute to be normal, and that less than 12 or more than 25 is considered abnormal (Cleveland Clinic Foundation 2014).

Chaitow et al. (2014) consider 10–14 breaths per minute normal with a 1:1.5–2 ratio of inhalation to exhalation. While the number of cycles per minute may be debatable, the ultimate goal of breath training is to improve the efficiency of one's breathing strategy, and to reduce the number of breaths per minute to a value closer to the lower end of the normal range (Osar 2015).

There are certain characteristics which indicate that the individual is using an optimal three-dimensional breathing strategy.

Ideally during inspiration:

- the diaphragm contracts (moves inferiorly from its dome shape), pushing the internal organs down toward the pelvis—there is a subsequent expansion in the entire abdominal and pelvic cavities;
- there is lengthening of the abdominal wall and pelvic floor;
- the scalenes contract to elevate the upper ribs;
- contraction of the sternocleidomastoid lifts the sternum and clavicles superiorly and anteriorly;
- the serratus posterior superior elevates the posterior aspect of the upper rib cage;
- contraction of the intercostals and levator costarum muscles elevates and posteriorly rotates the upper and middle ribs, increasing the intercostal spaces (the spaces between the ribs);
- the lower ribs expand laterally, but remain in a relatively low position;

- the serratus posterior inferior expands and stabilizes the lower ribs;
- the spine lengthens (relative extension), and the psoas stabilizes the trunk, spine, and pelvis.

The net result of these actions is an increase in the dimensions of the thoracic and abdominal cavities, which serves to expand and fill the lungs.

Ideally during expiration:

- the sternum and clavicles lower;
- the ribs move back to their resting position, and the intercostal spaces narrow;
- there is an elastic recoil of the lungs, diaphragm, pelvic floor, and abdominal muscles—the diaphragm and pelvic floor simultaneously move superiorly and return to a more domed shape;
- the spine gently flexes, but remains stable—the psoas likely contributes to controlling the degree of flexion that is occurring.

These changes decrease the dimensions of the thoracic, abdominal, and pelvic cavities to facilitate the release of air from the lungs.

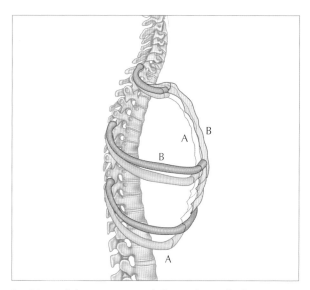

Position of the sternum and ribs at the end of exhalation (A); with inhalation both the sternum and ribs elevate to increase the anterior to posterior dimensions of the thorax (B).

Quiet, or resting, breathing should generally occur in a gentle wavelike motion. During inhalation, the chest and then the abdomen will rise, while during exhalation, the abdomen will gently lower, followed by the chest and thorax. During inspiration, the pelvis should gently widen as the organs descend and the pelvic floor eccentrically lengthens; during exhalation, the pelvis narrows as the organs rise as a result of the elastic recoil of their fascial attachments, and because of the elastic recoil of the abdominal and pelvic floor muscles.

Retraining Three-dimensional Breathing and TPC Stabilization

While three-dimensional breathing should be trained in a variety of positions, the supine position is the easiest and most preferred for the majority of individuals. The supine position with the legs supported over a chair or coffee table, and/ or with the feet resting upon the wall, offers several benefits, including:

- The position allows the body to be in an overall relaxed state.
- Lying with one's back upon a surface provides kinesthetic feedback from the posterior aspect of the body (head, trunk, spine, pelvis, and hips).
- Because the effects of gravity are minimized, it is the easiest position from which to educate and train neutral alignment of the head and neck, trunk and spine, and pelvis and hips.
- It is the most convenient position for incorporating movement of the arms and legs with breath and core training.
- Contact with the surface provides immediate feedback as to the position of the body.

For most individuals, their current breathing strategy is a result of a learned behavior; in other words, it has become their habitual pattern. Clinically, one of the most effective strategies for improving one's breathing strategy has been to:

1. Make the individual aware of their current strategy.
2. Educate the individual as to what a more optimal strategy looks and feels like.
3. Encourage the individual to maintain a regular and mindful practice schedule.

If your client struggles to achieve an optimal breathing strategy, or is experiencing discomfort in the supine position, try the prone, quadruped, side lying, and/or seated positions. Use the position(s) that best supports your client's ability to achieve the most successful three-dimensional breathing strategy. Ideally, three-dimensional breathing should be trained in all positions.

For the majority of individuals, breath retraining will be performed while inhaling through the nose and exhaling through the nose and/or lightly pursed lips. Inhaling through the nose has several benefits over mouth breathing, including:

- Filtering, moistening, and warming the incoming air.
- Providing greater resistance and a longer passageway to the lungs than with mouth breathing; this slows the breath rate, thus reducing the number of breaths per minute.

There is evidence that the floors of the mouth and tongue are neurologically linked with the pelvis, and are ultimately involved in breathing (Bordoni and Zanier 2013). When breath training is performed, the tongue should be positioned so that it is relaxed on the floor of the mouth (Osar 2015). During higher level or strenuous activities, it may be beneficial to have the tongue positioned behind the upper teeth, as a 30% increase in muscle activity using this tongue position has been found, compared with either placing the tongue on the hard palate or resting it on the floor of the mouth (di Vico et al. 2013).

Developing Neutral TPC Alignment

Achieving and controlling neutral alignment of the TPC is an important component of joint integrity as well as of overall health of the soft tissues. Neutral alignment is one of the easiest positions to achieve in order to support joint *centration (the optimal resting and loading position of a joint)*, to provide ideal proprioceptive feedback to the central nervous system, and to minimize wear and tear upon the joint and soft tissue structures.

Neutral alignment of the pelvis consists of an anterior pelvic tilt, with the anterior superior iliac spine (ASIS) slightly in front of the pubic symphysis. It is also important that there is control of both the lateral tilt and the rotation of the pelvis, so that it is symmetrically positioned over the femoral heads. A neutral alignment allows us to load the pelvis, as well as the hips and spine, so that there is the right amount of stress in exactly the right places across these joints. While it is impossible to maintain 100% of the time, the more time individual's spend out of their neutral alignment, there is an increased likelihood for wear and tear across the joints and soft tissue structures of the pelvis, hips, and spine. This is one of the mechanical factors that contribute to the degenerative joint process (Osar 2015).

Achieving neutral alignment of the pelvis and being able to optimally use the psoas also helps maintain neutral alignment of the lumbar spine— here, neutral alignment refers a slight lordotic curve. Since the psoas is the only muscle attaching directly to the front of the spine, it is a key muscle in maintaining this curvature. Maintaining the optimal position of the pelvis and lumbar spine will help an individual hold their posture and move without overloading the spinal, pelvic, and

hip joints in a manner that would otherwise create a wear and tear stress upon these regions.

Finally, the control of neutral pelvic alignment keeps us from having to compensate and overuse other muscles for support. When individuals lose neutral alignment, they will need to compensate by overusing certain muscles, which in turn contributes to chronic tightness. In fact, these compensations that hold the body in a non-neutral alignment are one of the most common causes of chronic tightness; for example, if the psoas and muscles of the DMS are not functioning as they should, it is common to overuse the superficial erector spinae, hip flexors and/or hamstrings to stabilize the spine and pelvis.

The Happy Baby position (see Chapter 3 for more on this) with the legs supported is one of the most effective ways to train neutral TPC alignment as well as three-dimensional breathing. It is such a great position because it helps align the individual in a manner that promotes the use of their respiratory muscles—primarily the diaphragm, intercostals, transversus abdominis, and pelvic floor. Actually, it is called the Happy Baby position because it is one of the earliest positions in which babies develop optimal breathing and core stability (image below). However, if the individual cannot lie comfortably on their back—in these cases, try the prone (stomach) position, or take them through the process while sitting in a chair or with their back against a wall. The breathing instructions will be relatively the same regardless of the individual's position.

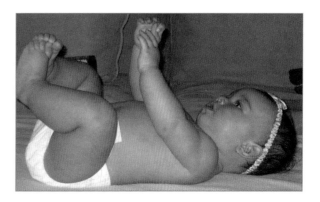

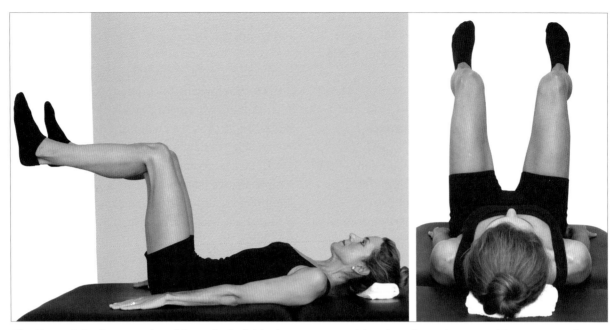

The Happy Baby Supported position—the individual assumes a position that allows them to achieve as neutral of a position as they are able.

The Happy Baby position, especially when combined with three-dimensional breathing, is one of our most effective methods to begin training more ideal postural alignment. Essentially, the individual is aligned in the relative position that they should achieve when they are in the upright position.

The first objective is to properly align the body, with the end goal being to align the TPC (i.e. the thorax is aligned over the pelvis, with neutral curves of the spine) so that the individual can properly access and incorporate the entire thorax, spine, and pelvis in the breathing process. This alignment will also relax many of the superficial muscles, making it easier for the individual to access the diaphragm and other primary respiratory muscles.

Please note: Do not force the individual into a specific alignment in an attempt to achieve more 'ideal' alignment. Many individuals will have adopted postures and spinal alignments to reduce stress upon their spine and neural structures (spinal cord, nerves, etc.). For example, individuals with spinal stenosis will adopt a more flexed lumbar

spine position and posterior pelvic tilt and therefore should not be forced into postures that compromise their neural structures. The most important goal when helping individuals develop a more optimal postural strategy is to help them make their overall alignment easier to maintain (i.e. reduce effort as well as potential wear and tear) and improve their ability to breathe three-dimensionally. Therefore the goal is to help each individual achieve their most neutral alignment or the position where they can be most relaxed and aligned. See Addendum on posture for more on this topic.

Pelvic Tilt

The Pelvic Tilt pattern, also referred to as an *Articulating Bridge* pattern, is one of the go-to exercises for developing awareness and training control of neutral TPC alignment. Although the focus is on the anterior and posterior motion of the pelvis, the pattern will also develop control over lateral tilt and rotation of the pelvis.

The Pelvic Tilt helps to train the muscles that control motion of the pelvis. Because the

Clinical Consideration

The anterior tilted pelvis is the position that will be used as the 'neutral' or starting position for most exercises in this book. The anterior tilted position of the pelvis is the position that best supports the lordotic curvature of the lumbar spine as well as a centered hip position. The ability to anteriorly tilt the pelvis and maintain neutral lordotic curve of the spine is one of the most effective strategies for effectively loading the posterior hip complex and reduce the risk of injury to the lumbar spine.

More important than the actual position of the pelvis and lumbar spine is the strategy the individual uses for posture and movement. If the individual is able to anteriorly tilt their pelvis and maintain a fairly lordotic curvature during most loaded exercises then the focus of their program is on their movement patterns and not creating an 'ideal' posture. However, if the individual has a non-optimal strategy for movement, for example, they are in a posterior pelvic tilted and lumbar spine flexion and maintain these positions during

their squat, deadlift, or other upright patterns, then the goal will be to help them develop a more anterior tilted pelvic position so they are able to appropriately load their posterior hip complex and minimize risk to their spine.

Because of the seated posture and focus on cues that have individuals 'pull in your abs' or 'squeeze your glutes', it is far more common that individuals with chronic hip and low back dysfunction present with posterior pelvic tilt and lumbar spine flexion. Some individuals will assume a posterior tilted pelvic position and lumbar flexed position to reduce neural stress (irritation to the spinal cord, nerve roots, and/or dural sheaths). The goal when working with these individuals is to help them lengthen and decompress their spine rather than trying to force them into an anteriorly tilted position.

See Addendum on posture for more on this discussion.

individual is supine, the effects of gravity are much reduced; this makes it easier for them to relax if they suffer from chronic tightness or gripping. They will also gain kinesthetic feedback from the floor, and it will be easier for them to make adjustments to their movement.

During the pattern, the individual will be able to relax many of the superficial muscles around the TPC, so that they will be better able to engage their psoas in its role of helping to achieve the neutral alignment of the pelvis and lumbar spine. The Pelvic Tilt helps to release chronic tension around the pelvis, spine, and hips, which further increases the individual's awareness of their position and movement.

While the psoas may be involved with the actual tilting of the pelvis, it plays a much larger role in this exercise by stabilizing the pelvis, spine,

and hips so in effect, the larger muscles—such as the superficial erector spinae, abdominals, hip flexors, and hip extensors—can move the pelvis with control. In turn, the Pelvic Tilt pattern helps mobilize the spine, which can help release chronic restrictions in those individuals experiencing true psoas hypertonicity (tension).

Setting Up the Pelvic Tilt Pattern

- Begin by having your client lie in the hook lying position—the hips and knees flexed, with the feet flat on the floor and about hip-width apart. The arms should be lying comfortably at the sides with the elbows flexed (image top left overleaf). In the case of an individual with increased cervical extension and/or suboccipital extension, place a small towel underneath their neck and head.

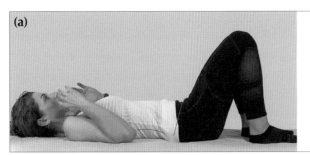 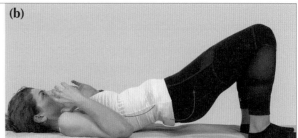

Neutral alignment—slight anterior pelvic tilt and lumbar lordosis; this is the beginning (a) and ending (b) position of the pattern. (b) Posterior rotation of the pelvis and reversal (flexion) of the lumbar curve.

- The pattern begins by performing short-range pelvic tilts—a posterior tilt by rocking the pelvis back (image below), followed by an anterior tilt to bring the pelvis forward. This movement should be easy and not forced.

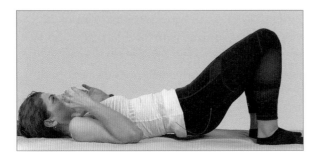

Posterior pelvic rotation and the beginning of lumbar spine flexion.

- As your client begins to release myofascial tension they will gain greater range of motion. They will begin to increase their posterior pelvic tilt and proceed to segmentally flex their lumbar spine (*segmentally* referring to the movement of one vertebra or segment of the spine at a time, followed by the next, etc.); this is often referred to as imprinting the spine into the surface (image above right). They continue to flex, or imprint, their spine as far as they are able. Your client should focus on releasing or lengthening through the front of their spine— essentially, the psoas should be lengthening at this point.
- The client reverses the pattern and slowly starts segmentally extending, or lifting, each vertebra off the surface and then rotating the pelvis back to the neutral, or anteriorly tilted,

position. It is at this point in the exercise that the psoas should become more involved in the motion. The client should imagine the psoas gently suspending or lifting the spine off the floor and pulling the pelvis gently down toward their feet.

The Pelvic Tilt pattern should be performed very purposefully, meaning that the individual should move attentively and with the intention of creating smooth, coordinated motion. The exercise helps to set up neutral and more relaxed alignment of the pelvis and lumbar spine; once this alignment is established, the individual integrates three-dimensional breathing.

For demonstration of the Pelvic Tilt pattern, visit www.IIHFE.com/the-psoas-solution.

Common Signs of Dysfunction in the Pelvic Tilt

Three common issues that can present during the Pelvic Tilt exercise are:

1. *An inability to achieve anterior pelvic tilt.* Since many individuals sit for a living, they are stuck in a position of posterior pelvic tilt and lumbar spine flexion. They often compensate for this posture by overlifting their rib cage or extending at the TLJ; this will make it challenging to shift the pelvis into an anterior pelvic tilt, which is the position we are ultimately trying to get the client to achieve.

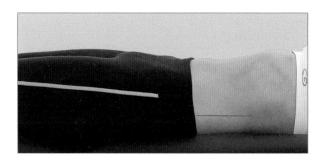

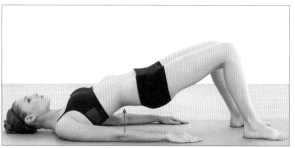

Thoracolumbar hinge—when the individual does not continue to articulate her spine she will begin overusing her erector spinae and extend at the thoracolumbar junction—note the spinal extension and resultant rib cage flare.

The client in the image above presented with chronic low back pain; she is a posterior hip gripper and is in posterior pelvic tilt (pubic symphysis anterior to the ASISs) and lumbar spine flexion while standing as well as when lying supine. Initially she found it challenging to rotate her pelvis anteriorly without compressing and irritating her lumbar spine. These individuals will often require myofascial release and cueing to release out of their gripping habits.

a. Have the client use myofascial release and/or trigger tools to release areas of chronic gripping—the posterior hip rotators, hamstrings, and abdominals will all pull the pelvis into a posterior pelvic tilt and inhibit any efforts to achieve an anterior tilt.

b. Cue the client to consciously let go of chronic gripping, and/or use manual release, foam roller, or trigger point tool to release chronic erector spinae muscle activity, before repeating the pattern.

2. *Thoracolumbar hinge.* A thoracolumbar hinge, or overactivity and gripping of the thoracolumbar erector spinae muscles at the TLJ (the area where the thorax joins the lumbar spine), will be common in many clients. The lumbar and thoracic erector spinae muscles cross the TLJ, and when the individual overuses these muscles rather than their psoas and multifidi in spinal stabilization, the erectors will pull the lower thorax and upper lumbar spine into excessive lordosis (see image above right). Releasing erector spinae activity can help improve someone's ability to activate their psoas. One sign of improved activation of the psoas is that the individual will move through the thoracolumbar region more fluidly and will be able to achieve a smoother lumbar curve, rather than just hinging or arching at the TLJ.

a. Have the client take 3 deep breaths in, focusing them into their belly and low back.

b. Have the client slowly and segmentally roll through that region to help reduce myofascial tone.

c. Use myofascial release with a foam roller or trigger point tool to release chronic erector spinae muscle activity in that region, and then repeat the pattern.

3. *Discomfort.* Never allow the individual to work through pain. If pain occurs in either extension or flexion, then decrease the range of motion and/or use myofascial or trigger point release on the hypertonic tissues, before repeating the pattern. If there is pain in both the flexion and the extension phases of the pattern, stop immediately and refer your client to a chiropractic physician or physiotherapist for a consultation, as this suggests a joint- or disc-related issue, which can be exacerbated through exercise.

Pelvic tilts performed in the upright position help develop the awareness and control to achieve neutral alignment. This is an important part of educating the starting and ending positions of most of the upright patterns that will be

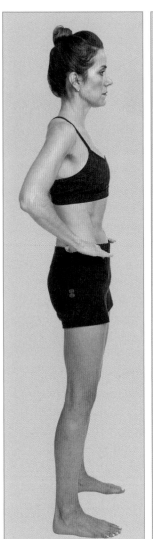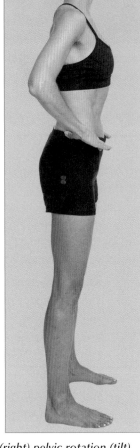

Posterior (left) and anterior (right) pelvic rotation (tilt).

discussed later in this book; squats, deadlifts, hip hinges, etc.

The individual places her hands upon her iliac crest (top of pelvis) with her thumbs towards the back and the fingers towards the front. She will use her abdominals and hamstrings to posteriorly rotate her pelvis (image above left) and then reverses the position to move towards an anteriorly rotated position (image above right). Ideally she'll end up closer to an anterior pelvic position. However, more importantly, the individual will assume the position that allows them to be most relaxed without placing stress upon her soft tissue and/or joints.

Developing Three-dimensional Breathing

Once the individual has found their best neutral alignment, they can begin training three-dimensional breathing to help coordinate the activation of the DMS with the regulation of internal (intra-thoracic and intra-abdominal) pressures.

Setting Up Three-dimensional Breathing

- The individual begins by lying on their back—preferably on a firm surface—with their legs supported over a chair or coffee table, or with their feet supported on the wall, about shoulder-width apart. The hips, knees, ankles, and feet should lie in parallel vertical planes, about shoulder-width apart. In this position, the individual should be as relaxed as possible.
- The individual's alignment should be as neutral as possible. Neutral alignment is where:
    - The head is aligned in such a way that a straight line passes from the top of the orbit to the mandible. If necessary and it is within your scope of practice, you can gently traction the head superiorly, and place a towel under the occiput and/or cervical spine to bring the head and neck into alignment.

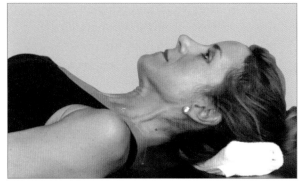

A towel or bolster can help position the head or neck in a more neutral alignment.

- The natural curves of the spine are maintained—cervical and lumbar lordosis, thoracic kyphosis. The ribs should angle slightly down so that the lower opening of the rib cage face towards the feet rather than towards the ceiling and the back of the neck is long (arrows in image below). This position helps promote the 'long spine' position that will be discussed throughout the book.

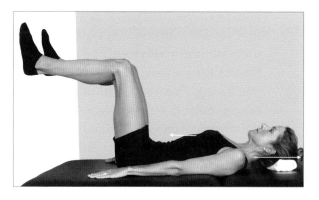

- The pelvis is in an anterior pelvic tilt. Have the individual perform pelvic tilts as discussed above and allow their pelvis to come to rest as close as possible to their neutral alignment (where the ASIS is slightly anterior to the pubic symphysis). Remember not to force this position.
- Breath training begins with focusing the breath in three distinct regions: abdominal, lateral (using the anterior rib cage from the first through the twelfth ribs), and anterior-to-posterior (again using the entire thorax from between the scapula through the lumbar spine). To retrain three-dimensional breathing, it is generally best to begin focusing on one region at a time. The greatest amount of time should be devoted to the area that the individual finds the most challenging, rather than trying to target all three regions at once.
- During quiet respiration, inhalation will occur through the nose, and exhalation will occur through pursed lips. The respiratory cycle should be made as effortless as possible,

and there should be no exaggerated or forced breaths. The focus will be on exhaling for twice the length of time taken for an inhalation; for example, if the inhalation lasts 3 seconds, the individual should work towards a 6 second exhale. To slow down the respiratory rate and allow more of a reflexive breathing pattern, a pause should be included directly after the inhalation phase of the pattern, as well as after the exhalation phase.

- Abdominal breathing: the individual places their fingers inside their ASISs to monitor for abdominal expansion during inhalation (image below). Taking a gentle breath in through the nose, they should feel the abdominal wall lightly push out into their fingers when there is adequate inferior movement of the diaphragm. Upon exhalation, they should feel their fingers sink back into the abdominal wall. There should also be a sense of the lower thorax and pelvis remaining in contact with the surface throughout the respiratory cycle, indicating optimal psoas stabilization of the lumbar spine.
- Lateral breathing: the individual places their hands on either side of their thorax or fingers just under their lowest ribs to monitor for lateral rib cage expansion

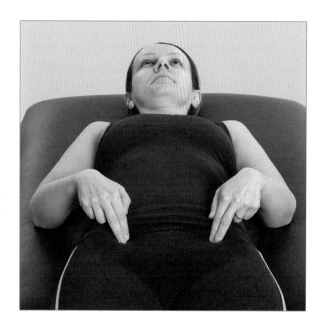

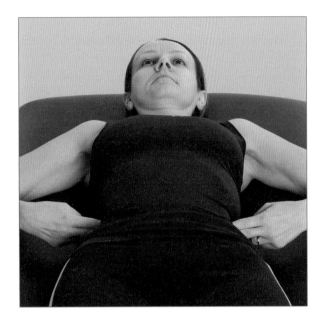

during inhalation (image above). When a gentle breath is taken in through the nose, they should feel the entire lateral aspect of the thorax expand lightly into their hands. As they exhale, the rib cage should return to its resting position.

If it is a struggle to achieve rib cage expansion, the individual can lightly squeeze their rib cage with their hands to kinesthetically cue breathing into that region of the thorax. They should release the pressure as soon as they feel the breath expanding the thorax beneath their hands.

During expiration, it is common for many individuals to find it difficult to get their thorax to move inferiorly. To assist the inferior migration of the thorax, they can lightly traction the rib cage down toward their pelvis as they breathe out, and then lightly hold it in this position as they take the next breath in.

- Anterior-to-posterior breathing: to facilitate anterior-to-posterior breathing, or expanding the thorax from front to back, the individual keeps their hands upon either side of their thorax or places one hand upon their chest and one upon their abdomen (image below). They should focus on the posterior (back) side of their thorax—visualizing and feeling their ribs against the surface. During the breathing cycle, they should visualize opening their posterior ribs with each breath in and allowing the rib cage to gently drop inferiorly on the exhalation.

Because they cannot see it, and have in all likelihood rarely thought about it, many individuals struggle in expanding the posterior aspect of their rib cage. If they have trouble with posterior expansion, they can wrap a bath towel or piece of elastic tubing around their rib cage and pull it snug. They should "breathe into" the towel or tubing, and then slightly release the tension as they breathe out, repeating for the desired number of repetitions. The prone position (Prone Lengthen) is another effective position for re-educating posterior breathing.

- Incorporating three-dimensional breathing: after having demonstrated proficiency in each of the three regions, the individual must be able to integrate them into a three-dimensional breathing strategy. Do not train three-dimensional breathing until you have first ensured that the individual has the ability to breathe in each of the three regions.

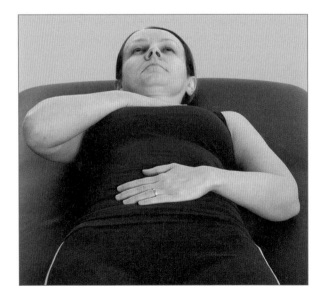

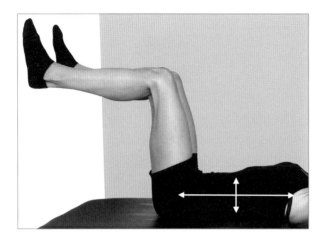

- The individual begins by breathing lightly in through their nose and out through their nose and/or through lightly pursed lips. The objective is to fill up the entire three cavities from top to bottom, side to side, and front to back with each inspiration (image above). The inhalation is followed by a light exhalation for approximately twice as long.

- As mentioned previously, it is very common for individuals to breathe far too fast and frequently, because of joint and myofascial restrictions, improper use of the DMS in stabilization, and habitual patterning. One of the most effective ways of achieving a more relaxed, fuller, and slower—in other words, a more efficient—breathing strategy is to perform the breath cycle in the following sequence:

  ▪ Inhale for 2 seconds, followed by a 1-second pause.

  ▪ Exhale for 4 seconds, followed by another 1-second pause.

  ▪ Repeat for another breathing cycle. Using this breath strategy, the individual will take approximately 8 seconds per breath or 7–8 breaths per minute—well within the desired range. The pause before and after each inhalation is effective for slowing down the rate and frequency, as well as for supporting a strategy that overall will be less effortful.

While making this change will initially be challenging, it is no different than training to run one's first 5K or trying to set a personal record in the weight's room. The individual should understand the importance of breath training to their overall health, and they must work at developing a successful strategy. To make this process efficient and rather effortless, they will want to be purposeful and persistent with the exercises, to allow successful integration of the strategy into their daily life.

After having established a more efficient strategy, the individual must be able to breathe in this manner in a variety of positions. With breath training, they must spend time consciously working on their breathing throughout the day as well as during their exercise program, so that they are able to integrate this new strategy; otherwise, they will likely fall back into their old breathing habits.

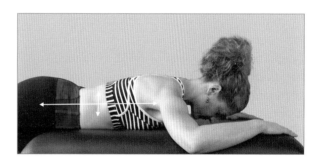

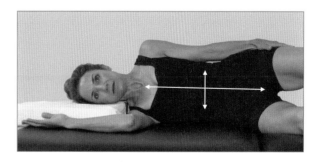

Three-dimensional breathing should be trained in a variety of positions including prone and side lying (images above). It is best to begin breath training under low loads and static positions

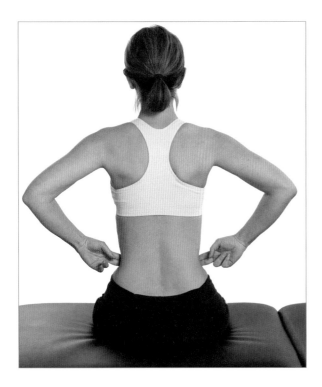

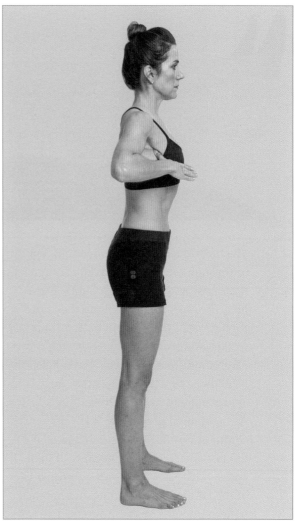

before incorporating it into higher level and dynamic activities.

To improve and incorporate it into upright positions and activities, individuals should be taught how to self-monitor for three-dimensional breathing. They can place their hands within their lateral abdominal wall (image above) or around their rib cage (image right) to ensure that each region of the TPC contributes to their overall breathing strategy. See Addendum on Suspension for more information regarding incorporating three-dimensional breathing into one's daily habits.

Important Note

When some individuals begin three-dimensional breathing, it is not uncommon for them to become light headed, as they are taking in much more oxygen, and letting go of more carbon dioxide, than they are used to. It can also occur if the individual is either forcing or rushing their breath—performing it too shallowly and

rapidly—and when the pause after each breath is too short.

To correct this, have them take a break from the new breathing strategy for that session, and allow them to return to their normal breathing strategy. At their next session, make sure that they are breathing in through their nose and out through lightly pursed lips. Next, rather than 3–5 breaths at a time, have them perform 1–2 breaths while not forcing either their inhalation or their exhalation. In addition, the use of the 1-second pause after each inhalation and exhalation is effective in slowing their breathing rate. These corrective strategies will usually solve the problem; however, if the individual continues to exhibit the same symptoms of light-headedness, be sure to have them follow up with their medical professional in order to rule out any underlying issues.

Integrating and Coordinating the Pelvic Floor with Breathing

Integrating and coordinating the use of the pelvic floor with breathing is an important strategy for improving activity of the deep myofascial system (diaphragm, psoas, and pelvic floor connection). The following section was kindly provided by pelvic floor specialist and colleague Dr. Judy Florendo.

This is the most consistently successful method I use with my patients to improve pelvic floor function and I have been able to confirm this through the use of diagnostic ultrasound.

The key to gaining optimal control of the pelvic floor (PF) is through breathing. After I teach someone diaphragmatic breathing first, I then move on to the PF. With PF hypertension and/or pain problems, I cue them to inhale "all the way down into the pelvis." I use an analogy: imagine your pelvic floor is an elevator in a high-rise building. Your "elevator"—your pelvic floor—is stuck in the middle of the building. When you contract, it goes up a little, but when you let it go, it's not going all the way back down to the ground floor." It is imagery like this that really starts to change what happens with my patients with short, tight pelvic floors.

If the individual has trouble releasing their pelvic floor with just a diaphragmatic inhalation (and in many cases, after I have done internal work and stretching), I will instruct them to: "inhale diaphragmatically and simultaneously gently bear down (or push—whatever they understand best)", and feel how that causes the PF to push or bulge down into my hand.

To improve PF activation or contraction (note— this strategy is specific for individuals working with a pelvic floor therapist and who have been identified as having a pelvic floor issue): After someone is able to demonstrate diaphragmatic breathing I have them gently—not abruptly, and this is critical—exhale and "draw the PF up and in." If I am performing internal work, I will instruct them to "close around my finger and feel how it pulls up and in." Then I will use the cue: "after a diaphragmatic inhalation, exhale easily and at the same time (and I stress "at the same time"), contract (or lift, or draw up) your PF."

Common Breathing Dysfunctions

In this discussion, *breathing dysfunction* (or disorder) refers to strategies that an individual has developed secondarily to their habitual or learned breathing patterns, in addition to a true respiratory pathology such as asthma. The strategy for addressing each of these breathing disorders therefore involves re-education of the individual with regard to their breathing pattern. Many individuals will require soft tissue work—either manually or via self-myofascial release—to release myofascial restrictions, and/or joint mobilization to restore optimal joint motion. Once the soft tissue or joint restrictions have been released, the individual is then instructed how to restore a more optimal breathing strategy using the previously described methods.

There are several common breathing dysfunctions of note.

Belly Breathing

While the terms "three-dimensional breathing," diaphragmatic breathing, and "belly breathing" are often used interchangeably within the health and fitness industries, a predominant belly breathing strategy is considered non-optimal. Many yoga instructors, Pilates instructors, and personal trainers encourage their clients to perform abdominal breathing, or *belly breathing*, where the focus is primarily on breathing into and expanding the abdominal region. This implies that utilizing a belly breathing strategy naturally improves the individual's ability to properly use their diaphragm and decrease the activity in their accessory muscles, such as the scalenes and pectoralis minor. While it may be better than performing a strictly chest dominant breathing strategy, focusing solely on belly breathing actually creates additional non-optimal strategies as a result.

Myofascial or joint restrictions of the thorax lead to general rigidity of the thorax. These findings are extremely common in individuals who have spent a significant amount of time doing core strengthening exercises, in those who have had abdominal, pelvic, back or cardiac surgeries, and in individuals who are overly braced or guarded secondarily to stress and/or as a result of their learned habits. These restrictions limit an individual's ability to create three-dimensional expansion of the rib cage (Osar 2015). Stiffness or restrictions of the muscles, fascia, and/or spinal or thoracic joints can inhibit optimal expansion and elastic recoil, thereby disrupting the respiratory process (Osar 2015, Chaitow et al. 2014).

In these individuals, belly breathing becomes a non-optimal strategy, because the focus is not on incorporating movement of the entire thorax as part of the respiratory pattern. In fact, an increased focus on belly breathing without incorporating three-dimensional expansion of the thorax contributes to an inefficient control of intra-abdominal and intra-thoracic pressures (Osar 2015). This strategy then perpetuates thoracic rigidity, which will eventually compromise spinal and pelvic stability (Osar 2015).

Additionally, individuals who have over-focused on belly breathing tend to create a learned inhibition of the abdominal wall, likely because there has been such chronic overstretching of these muscles and their investing fascia (Osar 2015). This, along with the loss of proper thoracic

involvement in the respiratory process, results in a migration of the organs inferiorly, generally caused by the loss of organ suspension within the thoracic, abdominal, and pelvic cavities.

The effect is that the organs of the gastrointestinal region sink into the lower abdomen; this, combined with the overstretching in the abdominal muscles and fascia, results in a distended appearance of the lower abdominal wall. Often this abdominal distension is attributed to 'weak' abdominals. However, upon palpation, the lower abdomen in these individuals will feel firm or rigid—even while they are at rest and not actively tensing their muscles. This lower abdominal distension, or "pressure belly" (Dr. Linda-Joy Lee), is commonly related to non-optimal control of the thoracic rings (term coined by Dr. Lee to describe a left and right pair of thoracic ribs and their corresponding vertebrae) and by the resultant loss of optimal pressure regulation within the TPC (Lee and Lee 2014).

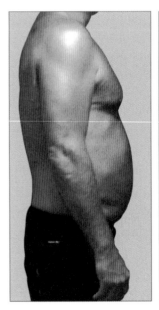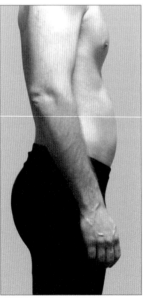

Lower abdominal distension and a resultant high level of resting tone in the abdominal wall will often be noted in individuals with non-optimal pressure regulation (images above).

Myofascial Restrictions of the Thorax

As noted above, myofascial restrictions of the thorax can put undue demands on the respiratory muscles and even alter their recruitment. Overactivity of the muscles around the thorax can challenge an individual's ability to breathe three-dimensionally and prevent the psoas from functioning optimally as a spinal stabilizer.

Some common areas of restriction are:

- *Abdominals.* The external and internal obliques have vast attachments to the anterior and lateral rib cage. When overactive, they will inhibit expansion of the rib cage during inspiration, and lead to a rapid expiration phase. The rectus abdominis has an attachment to the xiphoid process, and so shortness of this muscle will limit how much the sternum can elevate, thus limiting anterior rib cage expansion during inspiration. Overactivity and/or shortness in the abdominals will result in flexion of the lumbar spine, causing a decrease in lumbar lordosis, which in turn can lead to psoas inhibition (Osar 2015).

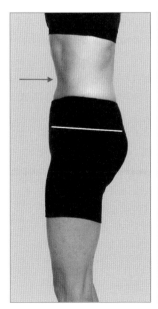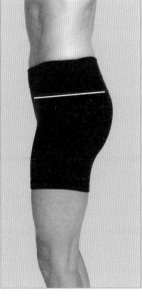

This patient presented with chronic low back pain and hip dysfunction. She is an abdominal gripper; note the hypertonicity of her abdominal wall which pulls her into a posterior pelvic tilt and lumbar spine flexed posture. This woman developed this posture after years of doing gymnastics during her teen years. One of the most important strategies for helping her decrease stress on her lumbar spine and to use her hips more appropriately when exercising was teaching her to relax her gripping strategy; note the improved alignment and pelvic and lumbar spine positioning when she relaxes her abdominal wall and posterior hip complex (image below left).

- *Erector spinae.* The erector spinae muscles run the entire length of the spine, from the pelvis to the occiput. When overactive, they will limit posterior expansion of the spine and rib cage. (The effect of overactivity of these muscles on the thoracic spine will be discussed further below.)
- *Latissimus dorsi.* Attaching from the lower thoracic and lumbar spine, thoracolumbar fascia, and pelvis, the latissimus dorsi inserts into the lesser tubercle of the humerus. When restricted, the latissimus dorsi will pull down on the shoulder girdle and/or cause extension in the TLJ; this will limit expansion of the upper, lower, or entire thorax during inspiration, and contribute to postural faults, including the forward shoulder posture and thoracolumbar extension.

Thoracolumbar Extension

Although the spine should lengthen (where *lengthening* refers to a relative extension of the spine) during inspiration, this should not be noticeable when observing an individual's breathing strategy. Individuals who do not have an optimal stabilization and three-dimensional breathing strategy will demonstrate increased thoracolumbar extension during inspiration. This is the common indication sign that the individual is not using their psoas appropriately to stabilize the TLJ.

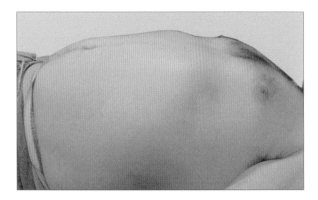

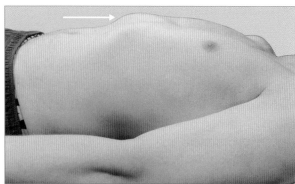

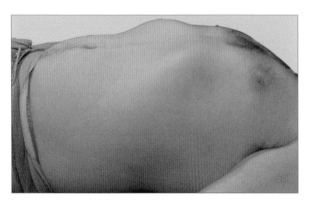

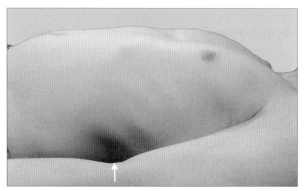

Inspiration (top image); Expiration (bottom image)— With general rigidity of the thorax (rib cage and spine) the individual is not able to fully utilize the entire TPC in his breathing strategy. He is a primarily an abdominal breather; note there is no inferior movement of the rib cage as he breathes out. This is a common breathing strategy with individuals that have chronic low back.

Additionally when the superficial erector spinae crossing the TLJ are overactive and/or the abdominal wall is inhibited, the abdominals cannot anchor the rib cage inferiorly during the respiratory cycle; this leads to flaring of the lower aspect of the rib cage, or causes it to remain in an inspiratory position during exhalation.

Rapid, Shallow Breathing

As discussed previously, rapid and shallow breathing is a telltale sign of a non-optimal breathing strategy. Similarly to what has been seen

Note the flared lower rib cage position during exhalation (horizontal arrow in top image) and the extension at the thoracolumbar junction during inhalation (vertical arrow in bottom image) in this patient with a history of chronic low back and hip pain. Increased thoracolumbar extension was palpated as he inhaled. This is a classic sign the individual does not have optimal spinal stability, and inspiration is causing excessive spinal motion.

in other muscles of the DMS, diaphragm function is affected in individuals suffering from chronic low back pain, as compared to individuals without low back pain (Bordoni and Marelli 2016, Vostatek et al. 2013). In individuals with chronic low back pain, the diaphragm was positioned higher in the thorax (a non-optimal resting inspiratory position), and breathing rate was faster and shallower, than in those with no low back pain.

Recall that this breathing strategy can directly contribute to a host of musculoskeletal and systemic issues, including chronic fatigue, muscle

Clinical Consideration

Those individuals who have sedentary occupations or spend long hours sitting have the perfect opportunity to practice their new breathing strategy throughout the day. They can set a timer on their computer, phone, or mobile device to go off every 20 minutes, for example, and then practice their new breathing strategy.

The individual stands up, aligns their posture (see Addendums on posture and sitting), and then squats back down onto the edge of the chair, perching themselves on their ischial tuberosities. They should focus on sending their breath, for 3–5 breath cycles, into the region(s) that are most challenging for them, and then return to their work. The entire process need not last longer than 2 minutes.

These periods of scheduled *micro-breaks*—short, regularly scheduled opportunities to work on posture, breathing, and/or corrective exercise—have made a difference for many patients, in terms of them being able to change chronic breathing disorders as well as postural dysfunction, muscle imbalances, and overall discomfort. The particular strategy described above is a go-to strategy for correcting TPC alignment, improving hip mobility, and maintaining optimal psoas function. It is particularly helpful for individuals experiencing chronic back or hip dysfunction.

The greatest benefit of these micro-breaks is that they are extremely effective in changing long-standing habits—those things individuals do almost unconsciously and are hardly aware of. Micro-breaks can be challenging for those with chronic issues, but when done mindfully, purposefully, and consistently, they are one of the most effective ways of changing non-optimal habits and adopting more optimal posture and movement strategies.

Summary of Psoas Function in Breathing

Psoas function at the trunk, spine, and pelvis
- Stabilizes the TLJ, lumbar spine, and pelvis to assist in maintaining TPC alignment during three-dimensional breathing.
- Functionally connects the diaphragm and pelvic floor, which likely facilitates coordinated activity between the two muscles.

Psoas function at the hip
- Centrates the femoral head within the acetabulum during breathing (although this function will become more predominant in the exercises covered in the next chapter).

weakness, and myofascial pain syndromes. Affected individuals need to be re-educated in how to slow their respiration rate while developing a more efficient breathing strategy. Releasing myofascial and joint restrictions, and then incorporating the deliberate 1-second pause after each inhalation and exhalation, has clinically been very effective in restoring ideal respiratory rates in these individuals.

Summary: Three-dimensional Breathing

1. The psoas has extensive fascial attachments to both the diaphragm and the pelvic floor. While not directly involved in the process, the psoas indirectly assists three-dimensional breathing by stabilizing the trunk, spine, and pelvis. It stabilizes the lumbar spine and pelvis to assist optimal function of the diaphragm and motion within the thoracic, abdominal, and pelvic cavities during the respiratory cycle. The psoas creates the appropriate amount of compression (stiffness) at the TLJ, so that breathing can occur three-dimensionally.

2. The psoas supports neutral TPC alignment and control, and neutral alignment and control of the TPC supports optimal strength and length of the psoas. The psoas helps support the TPC during the Pelvic Tilt pattern, thereby aiding in achieving and maintaining neutral alignment. Neutral alignment is the most optimal position for training three-dimensional breathing.

3. The psoas, as part of the DMS, promotes optimal stabilization of the trunk, spine, and pelvis, thus reducing the need for compensatory overuse or gripping within the superficial myofascial system (SMS). Three-dimensional breathing promotes optimal internal pressure regulation, and so there is less likelihood of overusing the SMS during trunk, spine, pelvis, and/or hip stabilization.

Thoracopelvic Cylinder (TPC) Stabilization

Anatomy of the Core

Most discussions about the body's core generally refer to the lumbar spine, pelvis, and hips, or the *lumbopelvic-hip complex*. Unfortunately, this viewpoint discounts the thorax's significant contribution as well as its direct impact on posture and movement. For a more holistic look into optimal core function as a necessary component of an individual's overall performance, a comprehensive approach must include the thorax. Therefore, going forward, any discussions of the *core* in this book will be referring to the entire thoracopelvic cylinder (TPC).

The TPC consists of the thorax (thoracic spine and rib cage), lumbar spine, and pelvis (image overleaf left). The hips, while directly impacting the TPC, are considered part of the extremities, and are thus not included in this view of the core. However, the TPC directly influences posture and movement of the head, neck, and upper and lower extremities, and is in turn influenced by these regions.

The TPC is referred to as a cylinder because the rib cage, sitting on top of the pelvis, forms a conceptual cylinder. The trunk muscles and fascia form the walls of this osseous, ligamentous, myofascial cylinder, while the fascial layers over the thoracic inlet and the pelvic floor form respectively the roof and the floor. Separating the thoracic and abdominal-pelvic cavities is the respiratory diaphragm; the psoas provides a direct myofascial link between the diaphragm and the urogenital diaphragm, or the pelvic floor (image overleaf right). The functional relationship between these structures was discussed in Chapter 1 (functional anatomy) and Chapter 2 (breathing).

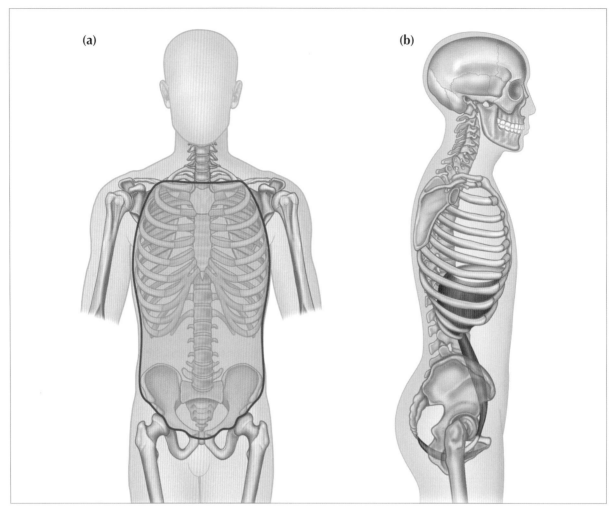

(a) The thoracopelvic cylinder (TPC); (b) the psoas is the myofascial link between the diaphragm and the pelvic floor and thus helps stabilize the TPC.

The TPC has a dual role in posture and movement. It has the unique ability to be highly stable and rigid for those activities requiring significant force production and/or reduction. Many activities—including lifting heavy weights, bracing for impact, and accelerating and/or decelerating one's body or an object—require immediate stability of the TPC to generate the necessary force to complete the task in hand and protect the multiple joints and internal structures contained within it. The unique feature of this cylinder is its ability to also be a mobile and adaptable structure for activities not requiring bracing, such as quiet breathing.

The TPC must also maintain its mobility and adaptability for the vast majority of activities in daily life, including postural control, rotation, and normal gait.

Regardless of the activity, the TPC must be able to appropriately adapt to the demands of the specific task, so that the task can be completed and the necessary protection for the joints and soft tissue structures can be provided. This ability to accomplish the demands of life, occupation, and sport while simultaneously providing optimal joint control is the next topic of discussion.

Developing A More Efficient and Optimal Strategy

When working with individuals that have chronic tightness, chronic pain, and/or the inability to perform at a level that they want or need, the initial focus of their rehabilitation and/or training program is to first assess to determine where there is a lack of efficiency and/or non-optimal strategies for posture and movement. The over-riding goal of their program then becomes to take this information and help them develop a more efficient and optimal postural and movement strategy so they can achieve their goal(s). The rehabilitation/training program, which may include but is not limited to strength, flexibility, coordination, balance, range of motion, mobility, etc., should assist them in using the least amount of energy or force to successfully complete the tasks within their program while also placing the least amount of wear and tear upon their joint and soft tissue structures as they work towards accomplishing their functional goals.

Core Stabilization

In the Integrative Movement System™ model, *core stabilization* is defined as the individual's ability to maintain the optimal TPC alignment, three-dimensional breathing, and appropriate levels of myofascial control required to efficiently complete the desired task. There are two terms—"efficient" and "optimal"—that really differentiate this definition of core stability. *Efficient* refers to using the least possible amount of energy for the task, whereas *optimal* refers to utilizing the most appropriate strategy for its successful completion.

An example of bending over to pick up a newspaper versus bending over to pick up a child will help illustrate this concept of core stability. Both movements require stabilization to control the trunk, spine, and pelvis as the woman bends

forward. However picking up the child requires a higher level of muscle activation to both complete the task and reduce the risk for soft tissue and/or joint injury.

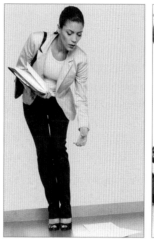 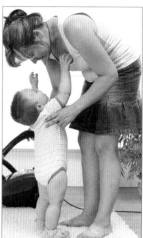

Any movement—bending included—requires a certain level of core stabilization to support, as well as to minimize the stress on, both the joints and the soft tissues of the trunk and spine. Bending forward to pick up a light object, such as a newspaper, should not require the same level of muscle effort as picking up a child. The core needs to be activated, because the joints and soft tissue structures need to be protected; however, a high-level bracing (co-activation of the core muscles to stiffen the trunk and spine) strategy should not be required to pick up the newspaper. On the other hand, picking up the child requires a greater level of joint control, and so a bracing type of contraction is more appropriate in this situation.

The important concept here is that in contrast to some industry methods, there should not be a universal, or one-size-fits-all, approach to stabilizing the core. The demands of life require that the intensity of core muscle activation be appropriate in order to safely and effectively complete the desired task. Problems arise when a bracing or high-level core stabilization strategy becomes an individual's default strategy in their daily life, because the ability to use the appropriate levels of control for the activity they are doing has been lost. Signs of this undesirable strategy will be discussed in the exercise section below.

Principles of Core Stabilization

There are three key principles to take into account when helping a client develop an optimal core stabilization strategy. These principles form the basis of the Integrative Movement System™ and are referred to as the *foundational ABC—* alignment, breathing, and control.

- *Alignment.* The individual must align and control their TPC. Optimal alignment of the TPC means that the thorax is stacked over the pelvis and that the spinal curves (cervical lordosis, thoracic kyphosis, and lumbar lordosis) are maintained. When the individual has optimal alignment, their joints are best positioned for loading and there is a decreased likelihood of incurring acute or repetitive trauma of the joints and soft tissues. The psoas, as part of the deep myofascial system (DMS), helps maintain alignment of the TPC in posture and in movement. The loss of ideal alignment compromises the individual's ability to activate their deep core muscles and to breathe three-dimensionally, which consequently affects both posture and movement (Osar 2015).
- *Breathing.* Three-dimensional breathing improves the use of the diaphragm, as well as the other respiratory muscles, in regulating pressures within the thoracic and abdominal cavities. It is the ability to regulate internal pressure that enables an individual to both stabilize and decompress their TPC. This dual ability to maintain stability without over-compressing their joints and spinal discs is truly one of the key features of three-dimensional breathing. It is also why many individuals who have focused primarily on using a core-bracing strategy will tend to over-compress their spine and increase the wear and tear on their joints and intervertebral discs. This is a common cause of degenerative joint and disc disease.

  Additionally, three-dimensional breathing helps activate the deep muscles (diaphragm, psoas, transversus abdominis, pelvic floor, etc.) that control the TPC (Osar 2015). When these muscles pre-activate prior to movement, they help stabilize the trunk and spine, so that the larger superficial muscles can do their primary jobs of moving the body and providing additional stabilization where necessary. In this relationship, three-dimensional breathing supports optimal function of the psoas; in turn, optimal psoas contribution in stabilizing the spine and pelvis supports optimal function of the diaphragm in three-dimensional breathing. Three-dimensional breathing also mobilizes the thorax, thereby relaxing over-contraction of the superficial muscles, such as the abdominals and erectors. Thus three-dimensional breathing promotes optimal stability as well as mobility of the trunk, spine, and pelvis.
- *Control.* After aligning the TPC and improving breathing, the individual must utilize their myofascial system (deep and superficial) to complete their functional tasks. It is important to note that, while the muscles of the deep myofascial system (DMS) can provide enough force to adequately control joint motion, they alone are not sufficient for providing the level of control required for most tasks in everyday life.

To adequately meet postural and movement requirements, there must be a balance between the deeper and more superficial myofascial systems. While muscles never work in isolation, there are inherent differences between the muscles that comprise the DMS and those that make up the superficial myofascial system (SMS); this will be the next topic of discussion.

Deep Myofascial System

As their name suggests, the muscles and investing fascia of the DMS are deeply located and tend to attach close to the joints; they fascially blend into the joint capsules and adjoining network of ligaments. Because the activity in these muscles needs to be more continuous, their fiber composition tends to be more oxidative in nature.

The muscles of the DMS have *feedforward* activity, meaning that they pre-activate or contract just prior to movement to stabilize and control joint motion. As these muscles also tend to have a higher percentage of proprioceptors, they are better able to detect and send messages back to the central nervous system regarding joint motion. The DMS is responsible for making minor adjustments, which facilitates efficient posture and movement. The psoas, along with the transversus abdominis, pelvic floor, multifidi, and diaphragm, is categorized as one of the muscles within the DMS.

Superficial Myofascial System

The SMS consists of the more superficial muscles and their investing fascia. The muscles within this system are fascially linked and form myofascial chains; it is these chains that are primarily responsible for movement and for providing higher levels of stabilization.

To illustrate the coordinated roles and use of the DMS and SMS, the example of bending down to lift a child will be used; this action requires

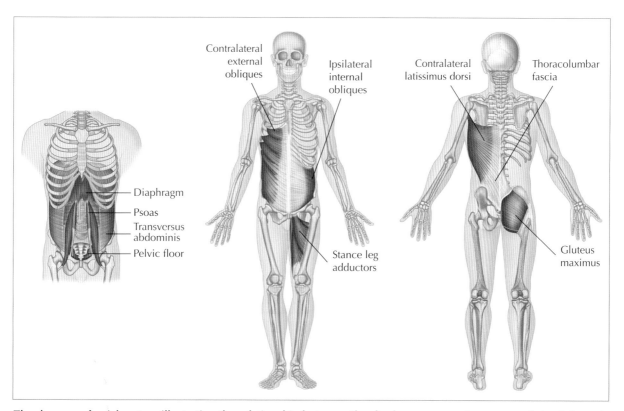

The deep myofascial system illustrating the relationship between the diaphragm, psoas, transversus abdominis, and pelvic floor (left); the anterior oblique chain (middle) and posterior oblique chain (right) are two examples of the superficial myofascial system.

TPC mobility and, naturally, a degree of stability. It is primarily the DMS that provides joint stabilization during bending, and there is light to moderate activity in the SMS to eccentrically control the movement and prevent overstretching of the soft tissue structures. Once engaged in the act of lifting the child, the SMS increases activity to stiffen the TPC, and, collectively with the DMS, serves a stabilizing function against the increased demands upon the joints and soft tissue structures.

In the aforementioned tasks, the TPC must be stable in order to support the load of the bodyweight and then the weight of the child, as well as the momentum involved with the activity. Had the individual just picked up a newspaper, however, a lower level of SMS activity would have been required for the task. This highlights the importance of having an efficient and optimal core stabilization strategy: it enables coordination of one's neuromyofascial systems and move efficiently between activities of different complexity, load, speed, and duration.

In this model there is a differentiation between tasks that require low levels of stability and those that require more moderate and higher levels of stability. While many tasks, such as lifting a child, will depend on one's overall strength and stability, there are certain tasks in life that should—in relatively healthy individuals—require a low-level stabilization strategy, and therefore more activity in the DMS and less in the SMS. Low levels of stability are required for tasks such as quiet sitting, standing, walking, bending, rotating, and breathing.

Higher levels of stability, and therefore higher SMS activity, are required for activities such as lifting, bracing for impact, and accelerating and/or decelerating the body or an object (throwing, punching, or kicking, and swinging a racquet, bat, or golf club).

Naturally, the levels of demand inherent in each task can vary. For example, a relatively lower level of stabilization is required during the backswing in golf (image below left). During the swing, or acceleration phase, there is a cascading demand, which peaks at the moment of impact with the ball (middle images below). Following the deceleration phase, the demand progressively ramps down, until the athlete returns to a more relaxed or low-demand state (image below right).

A summary of the two myofascial systems is provided in the table overleaf.

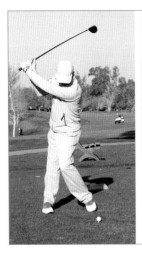 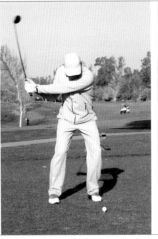 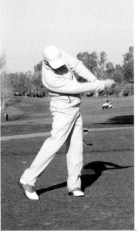 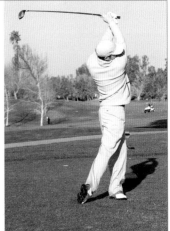

Comparison of the Characteristics of the Deep and Superficial Myofascial Systems of the TPC

	DMS	SMS
Size and location	Generally smaller muscles Located at deep to intermediate levels, connecting directly to, or near, the axis of rotation Generally connects intersegmentally (one joint segment to the adjoining segment)	Generally larger muscles Located at intermediate to superficial levels, connecting further away from the axis of rotation Generally crosses multiple joint segments
Fiber composition	Primarily type I, oxidative (use oxygen for energy)—fatigue resistant	Primarily type II, glycolytic (use glycogen for energy)—easily fatigued
Proprioception	Tends to contain a higher density of proprioceptors	Lower density of proprioceptors
Activation	Pre-activates prior to movement to provide segmental joint stability	Activates after the DMS to produce larger movements and higher levels of stabilization
Function	Specific control of joint position and motion Non-direction specific, meaning that the muscles activate regardless of the direction of movement	General, non-specific joint stabilization and movement Direction specific—muscles only activate as dictated by the direction of movement
Response to trauma, inflammation, or pain	Atrophy, timing delays, inhibition, decreased endurance, easily fatigable, decreased ability to control segmental joint position and motion	Hypertrophy, hypertonicity, lowered threshold of activation—results in increased resting joint compression and over-activity during low-level tasks
Muscles	Psoas, transversus abdominis, diaphragm, pelvic floor, multifidi (deeper fibers), quadratus lumborum (deeper fibers), intercostals, intertransversarii, interspinales, rotatores	Anterior and posterior oblique chain, lateral stabilization chain, deep longitudinal chain, superficial flexor and extensor chains

Note that some muscles (including the quadratus lumborum and multifidi) contain fibers that share characteristics with both categories; their deeper fibers tend to share characteristics of the DMS, and the more superficial fibers function more like those of the SMS.

Motor Control Training and Corrective Exercise

The overriding premise discussed in the previous section is that all activities in life require a certain level of TPC stability. What differs is the amount of stabilization and level of effort that is appropriate to the demands of the task. Problems tend to arise when the individual's core stabilization strategy is not adequate—i.e. not efficient and/or not optimal—for the demands of the task.

Research over the previous two decades has repeatedly and consistently demonstrated deficits—timing delays, decreased endurance, and atrophy—in the deeper core muscles (including the transversus abdominis, pelvic floor, multifidi, and diaphragm) of individuals experiencing low back pain (LBP) (Hodges et al. 2013, Hides et al. 2008, Richardson et al. 2004). Clinically induced muscle pain has been shown to create immediate changes in feedforward or anticipatory postural response of the trunk muscles (Hodges et al. 2003). MRI evidence has demonstrated that individuals experiencing LBP and sciatica tend to experience atrophy in their deeper muscles, including the psoas and the multifidi (Barker et al. 2004, Ploumis et al. 2011, Seongho et al. 2014). Additionally, breathing dysfunction, diaphragmatic fatigue, and proprioceptive deficiency of the diaphragm is noted in individuals experiencing chronic low back pain as compared to those not experiencing pain (Bordoni and Marelli 2016).

To compensate for the above-mentioned deficits, individuals will generally over-activate the SMS. For example, individuals with chronic LBP tend to demonstrate greater overall posterior oblique chain muscular activity (Kim et al. 2014) and greater rigidity with less variability in their gait, as compared with control participants (Lamoth et al. 2004).

Common clinical findings with individuals experiencing chronic hip and low back tightness or pain related to SMS overactivity include:

- Postural alterations (flared anterior ribs, overall thoracic rigidity in standing, hypertonicity of the spinal erectors in standing, overactivity of the superficial glutes in standing).
- Over-lengthening of the psoas on length assessment, and weakness during muscle testing.
- Non-optimal breathing strategy (short, shallow, and/or rapid breathing).
- Hypertrophy, as well as general overactivity, of the superficial abdominal and erector muscles during even low-level activities (e.g. sitting, standing, lifting something light off the floor, lifting a leg off the table or floor when supine).
- Bearing down (Valsalva's maneuver) and abdominal distension during trunk loading.

One of the most important methods for helping individuals improve function of the psoas and DMS and thus develop a more optimal posture and movement strategy is to incorporate the three key principles of the Integrative Movement System™—alignment, breathing, and control—into a corrective and functional exercise program. Utilizing these principles has been effective in improving motor control while consistently helping patients and clients work toward developing a more optimal postural and movement strategy, improve performance, and reduce symptoms related to chronic tightness and discomfort.

Motor control training—exercises and strategies focused on improving the activation, timing, duration, and specific joint control—as part of an overall training program is an important component in restoring balance between the DMS and SMS. Specific training of the muscles of the DMS has proved useful in reversing atrophy and reducing pain and disability in both the general population and high-level athletes experiencing low back pain (Hides et al. 2008, Hides and Stanton 2014, Hodges et al. 2013, Seongo et al. 2014). Research has also demonstrated that specific motor control training improves activation (timing) of the DMS in individuals with chronic LBP (Tsao and Hodges 2007), as well as in elite athletes with low back pain (Hides et al. 2016, Mendis et al. 2016). Interestingly, non-specific core training did not produce the same immediate effects as highly specific motor control training (Hall et al. 2009).

Clinical Consideration

One additional benefit of motor control training arises from the fact that many traditional rehabilitation and strength and conditioning programs predominantly focus on training the SMS relative to the DMS. Often the effectiveness of rehabilitation or training programs is based solely on whether or not the individual can lift more weight, perform more repetitions, and/or move faster than when they began the program. While necessary, these metrics are not accurate indicators as to whether or not the individual is actually performing their patterns with greater efficiency or reducing the risks of wear and tear upon their body. This is not to suggest that increasing strength should not be an important metric and goal of training. To be fair, monitoring and measuring an individual's improvement in movement quality tends to be more challenging and does require an advanced skill set. However, when working with individuals that are experiencing chronic tightness, chronic pain, or a loss of performance, the primary goal is to improve movement efficiency and to identify as well as where necessary modify non-optimal habits that are contributing to their issues. This is the primary reason for including a motor control component as part of a comprehensive corrective exercise and strength program in helping clients successfully overcome chronic issues related to quality of movement. Many of the strategies in this book are designed to help improve motor control as part of improving a client's overall movement quality.

When there is an imbalance between the two myofascial systems, unless the training specifically focuses on the DMS, the SMS will continue to dominate; therefore traditional training approaches continue to perpetuate (and can even increase) the dominance of the SMS (Osar 2015). Clinically, an imbalance between the DMS and the SMS is one of the most common contributors to a non-optimal core stabilization strategy, and to the occurrence of chronic back and hip tightness and/or discomfort. Motor control training thus becomes an especially important part of an overall program for individuals demonstrating imbalance between the DMS and SMS.

Although it is difficult and often times not practical to isolate a single muscle contraction, when motor control deficits (timing delay, atrophy, and/or fatigue) are present, specific isolation—or rather preferential recruitment—of the DMS is required in order to improve function. While many detractors of motor control training will suggest that it is impossible to 'isolate' muscles since the brain only knows movement, there is increasing evidence to suggest there are indeed benefits in improving functional outcomes and decreasing pain when using isolation or preferential recruitment of the DMS. In addition to the work by Hodges, Hides, and Richardson previously noted, specific focus on using the lumbar multifidi muscles showed better functional outcomes in individuals with low back pain as compared to those who performed a more general abdominal and low back strengthening program (Soundararajan and Thankappan 2016). Therefore, while there will be many references made to specific muscles such as the psoas or pelvic floor throughout the exercise sections of this book, the over-riding goal of the training strategies presented in this book is to create improved balance and coordination between the deeper and superficial muscles rather than simply attempting to 'isolate' certain muscles.

The Role of Motor Imagery and Cuing in Corrective Exercise

Training the deeper muscles is an important part of training because as has been discussed, in the presence of motor control deficits, there is a tendency for the individual to compensate and overuse the SMS thereby increasing its activity. This over-activity of the SMS often inhibits optimal activation of the DMS, making it challenging to change one's current habits and adopt a more optimal posture and movement strategy.

There are several methods that are effective in developing improved awareness and activation of the DMS. One method that demonstrates consistent clinical improvements in individuals with chronic non-optimal posture and movement habits is motor imagery. The Integrative Movement System Corrective Exercise Strategy™ (Osar 2015) incorporates motor imagery as a way of developing and training more optimal postural and movement strategies.

Motor imagery (also referred to as *mental practice* or *visualization*) is the process of using thoughts to simulate the successful completion of an action or movement of one's body. While it is commonly used to improve athletic and dance performance (Schuster et al. 2011, Franklin 1996), motor imagery is also extremely effective for activating the DMS and creating more efficient posture and movement patterns (Osar 2015). For dancers experiencing altered core muscle activity secondary to back pain, the technique has been shown to help improve their muscle activity to a level resembling that of dancers who did not have low back pain (Gildea et al. 2015).

Another method that is extremely beneficial in improving function of the DMS is cuing. Cuing is one of the most important strategies for connecting to the DMS, and thereby improving conscious awareness of one's postural and movement habits. While the ultimate goal of corrective exercise is to make the changes occur at an unconscious level, conscious attention to one's position, movement, and muscle activation during motor control training has proved to be effective in restoring timing delays of the DMS in individuals experiencing chronic low back pain (Hall et al. 2009, Tsao and Hodges 2007, Tsao and Hodges 2008).

The use of specific cuing to activate the psoas and the DMS will be incorporated throughout the exercises. There are four different types of learners and learning styles: (1) verbal (individuals who need to hear and understand the instructions); (2) visual (individuals who need to watch and see what the clinician or trainer wants them to do); (3) kinesthetic (individuals who have to actually do the exercise or need to have their body palpated in order to ensure that they are accurately creating the right alignment, breathing, or movement pattern); and (4) mixed (most individuals are a combination of two or more of the above types). Experiment with visual, verbal, and kinesthetic (tactile) cuing, and determine which one (or more) resonates and creates the most optimal response in your client.

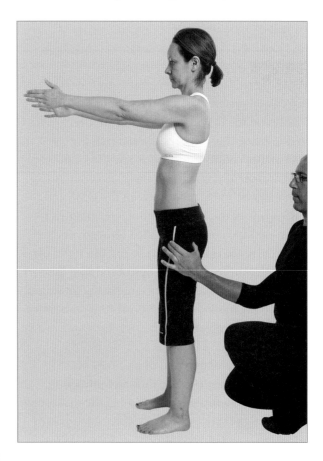

Examples of utilizing kinesthetic and verbal cuing: To improve hip hinging (image above) the individual's awareness is brought to her hip (femur) position relative to her pelvis. She is verbally cued to 'relax' her posterior hip muscles to reduce posterior gripping and to 'sit back' in her hip to encourage optimal hip hinging and bending patterns.

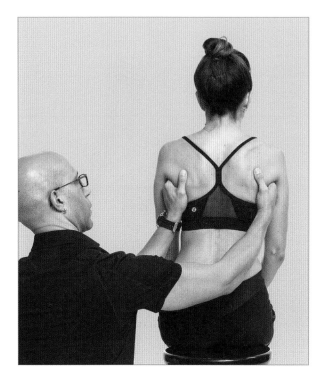

To decrease thoracolumbar extension and over-compression of the TPC secondary to over-activity of the erector spinae and/or latissimus dorsi, the individual is cued to 'create space between your ribs' or to 'suspend and breathe into your arm pit region' (image above). These are effective cues for individuals that experience chronic back tightness or discomfort when sitting, squatting, or deadlifting.

Additionally, the DMS tends to respond better to *internal cuing*, or verbal cues that utilize the brain to create awareness and to make connections to deeper regions and muscles of the body (Osar 2015, Osar and Bussard 2016). The SMS tends to respond better to action commands and external cues, such as "brace," "squeeze," and "harder" (Osar 2015, Osar and Bussard 2016). While external instructions and cues such as "explode off the blocks" have been shown to be superior in improving sport- or task-specific skills such as sprinting (Benz et al. 2016), clinical experience has demonstrated that external cuing less effective than internal cuing when trying to activate the DMS or in developing more efficient posture and movement. In individuals with chronic posture and movement dysfunction, internal cues tend to facilitate more optimal neuromotor connections, whereas external cues have a tendency to perpetuate the individual's habitual patterns.

The cues used throughout this book are modified adaptations learned from some of the best motor control teachers in the industry, including (but not limited to) Linda-Joy Lee, Ph.D., PT, Diane Lee, PT, Paul Hodges, Ph.D., Julie Hides, Ph.D., Carolyn Richardson, PhD., Gwendolyn Jull, PhD., and Sean Gibbons, as well as from industry colleagues Ed Flaherty, PT, CMT, Judy Florendo, DPT (pelvic floor specialist), Sara Fisher, CPT, IMS (former professional dance), and Jenice Mattek, LMT, IMS.

Important Note About Cuing

Take care to avoid over-cuing the individual: over-cuing can lead to frustration as well as unsatisfactory clinical results. While the correct cuing can be instrumental in activating a more optimal posture or movement strategy, too many cues can paralyze the individual. This can lead to the individual overthinking or over-processing and can actually worsen postural or movement patterns.

Choose one cue (or at maximum two) that best addresses the individual's primary issue; use that one as long as it works, but feel free to change and/or experiment with other cues as the relationship develops and the clinician/trainer gets a feel for how the client best learns and responds.

Cuing Activation of the DMS and the SMS

A comparison of the different cues for activating the DMS and the SMS is presented in the table below.

Cues to Activate the DMS and the SMS	
DMS	**SMS**
Responds better to verbal and visualization cues including:

"visualize," "connect," "feel," "imagine," "lighter" | Responds better to action or doing cues such as:

"contract," "brace," "squeeze," "harder," "more," "drive" |

Specific cues to activate some of the muscles of the DMS are listed below. Use pictures and/or models to educate clients and facilitate learning as well as awareness of these muscles. Because these muscles are deeper, generally harder to access, as well as there is relatively less awareness around them, be sure to get permission and it is within one's scope of practice when using tactile cuing or palpation techniques.

- *Psoas*
  - To improve spinal stabilization: "Imagine a wire connecting to the front of each vertebra in your low back. Now, without moving, imagine gently drawing that wire up toward your head."
  - To improve hip centration: "Imagine a wire connecting from the front of your spine to the ball (femoral head) in front of your hip joint. Now gently draw that ball into the socket (acetabulum)."
- *Transversus abdominis*
  - "Imagine your transversus abdominis is a layer of plastic wrap lying across your lower abdomen. Gently draw that wrap taut across your lower abdomen."

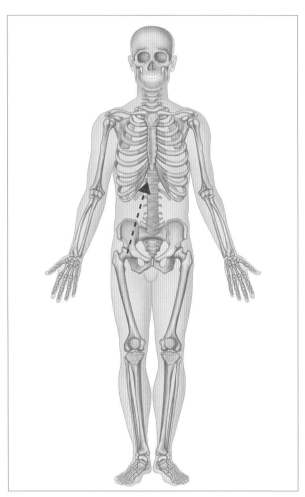

An effective cue for improving psoas activation is to imagine a wire connecting the hip to the spine and drawing the ball (femoral head) into the socket (acetabulum).

- "Imagine there's a wire connecting your left ASIS to your right ASIS. Gently tension that wire so that it lightly draws your ASISs away from each other."
- *Multifidus*
  - "Imagine there is a wire connecting the front of your abdomen to the back of your spine. Visualize gently drawing that wire toward your spine."
  - Palpation: the clinician places their fingers on either side of the spinous process, and cues the individual: "Gently fill up the space under my fingers" or "Connect a line from your transversus abdominis to my fingers and elongate through this level."

- *Pelvic floor*
  - General activation: the use of pictures can be very helpful, because this is a sensitive region, and often individuals are unfamiliar with the fact that there are muscles located here. The specific cues used most frequently for activating the pelvic floor while incorporating three-dimensional breathing were discussed in the breathing chapter.
  - Additional cues that we use with less frequency include: "Imagine a wire connecting from the pubic symphysis to your coccyx. Lightly tension that wire. Now breathe into that tension."
    For females: "Lightly tense your vaginal wall or perineum (area between the vagina and the anus). Now breathe into that tension."
    For males: "Lightly tense your perineum (area between the testicles and the anus). Now breathe into that tension."

Note: Although widely practiced, cues such as "imagine you are urinating, now try to stop that urine flow" are used with less frequency. After discussions with several pelvic floor therapists, they have suggested that these types of cue tend to overuse the wrong muscles and train a non-optimal response of the pelvic floor muscles. However, if a patient/client has been seeing a pelvic floor therapist and been given specific cues to use, continue with them. Allow the individual to keep using what they have been successful with, and/or what has been prescribed by their specialist.

Once a muscle has been activated, have the individual coordinate this isometric muscle contraction with three-dimensional breathing. This is an important part of developing coordination between respiration and muscle activation, as well as ingraining use of that muscle into the individual's neuromotor patterns.

Clinical Consideration

There has been debate as to the best method of cuing to improve performance. There is research that supports the use of external over internal cuing for improving performance, such as in sprinting or weight lifting (Benz et al. 2016).

Clinically there are benefits with utilizing the two types of cuing in both rehabilitation and training environments. While working with professional dance companies in Chicago for the past eighteen years, and while observing rehearsals, internal cuing was frequently incorporated. Sara Fisher, Certified Integrative Movement Specialist™ and former professional dancer, shares that the use of internal cuing has been instrumental since her early days of dancing in helping her make more powerful connections within her body. Nearly every dancer seen clinically has shared similar experiences of their own dance training.

So rather than debate which is the more effective type of cuing, find the best way to incorporate both types of cuing into a client's program. The following is an example of using both types of cuing in a corrective exercise and training program. While there are several different cuing examples, remember not to over-cue the individual. Choose one cue (or at maximum two) that works best for your client.

Example of cuing a client that has been experiencing chronic tightness and discomfort while running: Rachel is a 35-year old runner who presented with a non-optimal breathing strategy, and a poor ability to activate her DMS; she has instability when standing on one leg, and tends to overuse her SMS during low-level tasks, such as hip flexion while in a single-leg stance. When running she tends to hold her thorax in extension and tuck her pelvis into a posterior pelvic tilt.

These findings translate into some of the reasons why she is experiencing chronic hip and back hypertonicity, and self-reported decreases in her performance.

Following soft tissue release, she is cued to relax her SMS, using internal cues such as "let the tension go" or "soften your body." Next, she is taught three-dimensional breathing and psoas activation to improve hip dissociation, using internal cues such as "connect a wire from your spine to the front of your hip and then lift your leg off the table from that wire" or "float your leg off the table as you lift it up."

To prevent over-extension of her thoracic spine when she runs, she could be cued to "lengthen from the back of the head and keep the chest soft." As she lifts her leg, she is cued to "stay long through the spine," and visualize the psoas cue we used while on the table to help improve upright alignment and use of the psoas when in single-leg stance.

Upon being moved on to the treadmill to incorporate the earlier corrective exercise strategies into her running patterns, she is cued to maintain her spinal alignment with "keep your spine long and chest soft." Now that she has a better internal connection to her DMS, her focus will shift externally, where the goal will be to improve her running mechanics. A common external cue to improve both hip extension and foot turnover would be "drive your foot across the ground as if you are kicking up pebbles behind you from underneath your foot." Demonstrate this technique so that she has the correct visualization and is better able to accurately replicate the cues.

This an example of how both internal and external cues can be used to maximize what is being addressed from a corrective exercise standpoint, and how it can be incorporated into the functional movement patterns that clients and patients need and want to do.

Activating the Psoas

The psoas will be activated in a similar way to the rest of the DMS. There should be preferential activation of the DMS—for example, the transversus abdominis, pelvic floor, multifidi, and psoas—just prior to recruitment of these muscles' functional synergists—the external obliques, glutes, and iliacus. The goal during retraining is to preferentially activate the psoas, without simultaneously engaging the superficial hip flexors (rectus femoris and tensor fasciae latae) or the adductors.

- Lying supine with the leg over a stability ball or chair, the individual is cued to activate the DMS (use the most appropriate cue from the list above).
- With one hand, she palpates the front of her hip, to ensure that she is not activating the rectus femoris, tensor fasciae latae, or

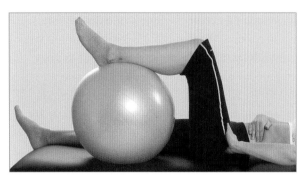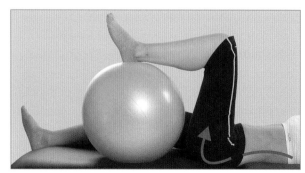

Psoas activation with hip flexion—The individual monitors that she is not over-using the superficial hip flexors as she is flexing her hip (left image) and maintains alignment of her spine throughout the pattern (right image).

adductors and to reduce overuse of superficial myofascial breathing. She should visualize a deep wire connecting the front of her spine to the front of her hip near the groin area where the psoas attaches to the lesser trochanter of the femur.

- Maintaining the activation of the DMS, she slowly rolls the ball or slides her leg along the chair (flexing her hip), and returns it to the starting position. She is drawing the knee in towards the trunk with a balance of the DMS and SMS.

She maintains activation of the DMS and practice three-dimensional breathing throughout the repetitions. She moves her leg through the range of motion that allows her to maintain psoas activation, with minimal to very light engagement of the superficial hip flexors. It is recommended to perform 5–10 repetitions for 2–3 sets. Once activated, the psoas must be coordinated into a core exercise progression that integrates its function with the rest of the deep and superficial myofascial systems.

For demonstration of Psoas activation, visit www.IIHFE.com/the-psoas-solution.

Psoas' Dual Role

As previously discussed, the psoas plays an integral role in stabilization of the TPC, as well as in alignment and control of the hips. Recall that the hips—the femoral heads and acetabula—are ball and socket joints and thus have a dynamic range of motion. While this design provides a certain level of inherent stability, myofascial control is also required in order to provide both static and dynamic centration for these joints. The psoas, as part of the DMS, provides a significant amount of this stability.

In the functional anatomy chapter (Chapter 1), it was discussed how the psoas centrates or maintains alignment and helps to control the femoral head within the acetabulum. During hip flexion, for example, the psoas centrates the femoral head within the acetabulum, so that the other hip flexors—iliacus, rectus femoris, tensor fasciae latae, and sartorius—can actually flex the hip. In this manner, the psoas helps ensure that hip flexion is smooth, coordinated, and efficient. The following series of exercise patterns will describe how to involve the psoas in its dual role of a TPC stabilizer and hip centrator.

Happy Baby

The Pelvic Tilt (Chapter 2) helps to increase awareness and control in achieving more neutral alignment of the pelvis and spine. Three-dimensional breathing helps improve the use of the diaphragm and other muscles of respiration. Because of its neural and fascial connection with the diaphragm, three-dimensional breathing helps activate the psoas in stabilization and control of the TPC. The Happy Baby pattern will introduce how to further incorporate the psoas into the stabilization of the trunk, spine, pelvis, and hips.

There are three primary ways in which the psoas contributes to optimal performance in the Happy Baby pattern:

1. The psoas helps stabilize and maintain lumbar lordosis, thus preventing either spinal flexion (flattening of the lumbar spine) or thoracolumbar extension as the hips are raised and lowered.
2. The psoas helps to maintain a neutral pelvic alignment (anterior pelvic rotation), thus preventing posterior pelvic rotation as the hips are flexed, and excessive anterior rotation as they are lowered.
3. The psoas and lower glutes help centrate the femoral head within the acetabulum; together, they ensure optimal hip flexion (hip hinge) and the maintenance of neutral pelvic and spinal alignment throughout the pattern.

In Chapter 2 the Happy Baby position with the legs supported was used to train three-dimensional breathing. The Happy Baby will again be used to further incorporate the psoas into the control of hip flexion. The goals of the Happy Baby with hip flexion pattern are threefold:

1. To train the psoas and DMS in the control of neutral TPC alignment while supporting a load—in this case the legs.
2. To coordinate activity of the DMS with three-dimensional breathing, and balance activity between the deep and superficial myofascial systems.
3. To train psoas activation in training hip dissociation—flexion as the legs are raised, and eccentric control as the legs are lowered—and shoulder dissociation in the Pull-over pattern.

Setting Up the Happy Baby Pattern

- The individual begins by lying supine, with their legs supported on a stability ball (image below), coffee table or chair, or with their feet flat upon the wall. They should be positioned as close to neutral as it is possible for them to achieve. Recall that neutral alignment is where the pelvis is in a slight anterior pelvic tilt, and the curves of the spine are maintained—the cervical and lumbar spines are lordotic, and the thorax is aligned with the pelvis. We do not want to see any changes in this TPC alignment at any point during the Happy Baby pattern.

- As mentioned in Chapter 2 in the Happy Baby with supported legs, clients with tight or restricted hips should be positioned so that they can achieve neutral alignment, which usually means they will have less hip flexion. Furthermore, some clients will need a bolster under their head and neck in order to bring them into better alignment with their trunk.

- Lifting one leg: once positioned, the individual begins three-dimensional breathing. Create a visual image for them about the location and function of the psoas. The cue used most often with clients is: "Visualize a wire attaching from the front of your spine to the front of your hip. Imagine that your leg is light and that you are lifting your leg from this wire."

  The individual lifts one leg up off the surface and brings it back down using the previous visualization. To improve eccentric control of the psoas, they are cued: "Keep your leg light,

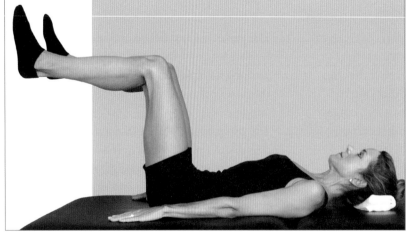 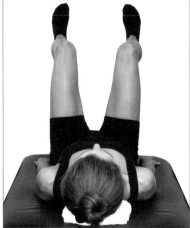

Happy Baby with feet supported upon wall—this is the preferred position of the pattern as the individual can position their hips about shoulder-width apart and will generally promote a relaxed position for the hips. The individual will also be positioned close to the wall so that their spine is in the most neutral position they can achieve; use a towel support to align the head and neck with the TPC.

and use the wire to bring your leg back down to the surface."

The sequence is repeated with the other leg, alternating the two sides until the individual has performed 5–10 repetitions per side with no compensations. Once they can do this pattern for a minimum of 5 repetitions per side without compensation, they can progress to lifting both legs.

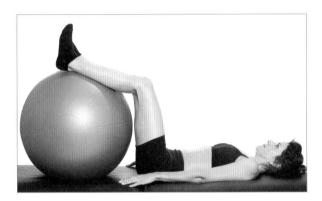

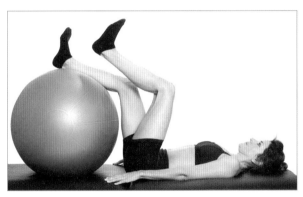

Happy Baby legs supported over stability ball—single leg lift.

- Lifting the second leg: using the same cues as above, the individual lifts one leg and then slowly lifts the second leg, so that both legs are unsupported. In this position they perform 3–5 diaphragmatic breaths and then bring their legs back down to the surface, one at a time. Again, there should be no change in the alignment of the spine, pelvis, or hips throughout the pattern. Some individuals

may only be able to perform one breath with the legs elevated—in this case, have them perform just a single repetition and gradually progress them to the point where they can perform the pattern with 3–5 diaphragmatic breaths.

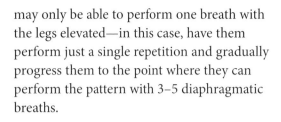

Happy Baby legs supported over stability ball—double leg lift.

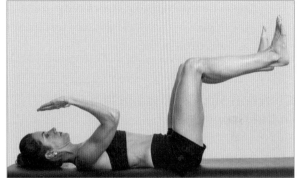

- Happy Baby unsupported (image above)— In this position the individual's head and neck are aligned with the TPC and the hips are flexed and about shoulder-width apart. The arms are raised so that the back of the scapula (shoulder blades) are in contact with the table. She should be able to maintain this position relatively effortlessly while maintaining three-dimensional breathing.

For demonstration of the Happy Baby pattern, visit www.IIHFE.com/the-psoas-solution.

- There are several ways to determine whether or not the psoas is activated, and whether or not the hip is remaining centrated as the individual is lifting and/or lowering their leg:
    - Note the amount of effort they are using—a well-centrated hip can be flexed without a lot of effort or gripping of their superficial hip flexors.
    - The pelvis and spine remain stationary as the hip is flexed.
    - The hip appears to drop posteriorly as the hip is being lifted, with no change in pelvic alignment.
    - Palpate and feel the hip sink into the acetabulum as the hip is brought into flexion.
    - Palpating the superficial hip flexors with one hand and the psoas (within the abdomen between the umbilicus and inguinal ligament) with the others, note activation of the psoas (tensioning under the fingers within the abdomen) just prior to movement of the leg.

Common Signs of Dysfunction in the Happy Baby

There are three common issues that present when clients perform the Happy Baby pattern. Primarily these relate to how the individual is compensating for the lack of psoas and deep myofascial control.

1. *Loss of neutral alignment.* The most common compensatory pattern is where the individual extends at their thoracolumbar junction (TLJ) and/or posteriorly rotates their pelvis and flexes their lumbar spine flexion. This is caused by non-optimal TPC stabilization and/or non-optimal hip dissociation (ability to move the femur independently of the pelvis). Notice changes in head, neck, and/or shoulder positioning because they are over-recruiting their spinal erectors and chest muscles for support.
    a. Cue the individual how to maintain control by thinking about the psoas as a wire connecting their spine to their hip. They will then lift and lower their leg using this wire connection.
    b. Have the individual breathe to gain control of internal pressure, and then repeat. Cue them to lift their leg on an inhalation, and lower it on an exhalation.
    c. Do not be afraid to regress the pattern. Since many individuals have become strong from using non-optimal strategies, have them begin by lifting one leg at a time, or simply sliding the leg rather than lifting it. Even just initiating hip flexion rather than actually lifting the leg can be an effective means of retraining psoas activation.
    d. Releasing chronic gripping around the spine, pelvis, and/or hips with a foam roll or through tactile cuing can also be helpful. For example, you can cue them to: "Let your ischial tuberosities (or sits bones) go wide" or "Imagine your hip joint is like a tire on an axle—the leg (tire) spins around the pelvis (axle) as you lift your leg."
2. *Abdominal distension.* The most common and indicative sign of a non-optimal core stabilization strategy is abdominal distension. The individual will bear down—essentially they are performing a Valsalva's maneuver—for TPC stabilization, rather than being able to use an optimal internal pressure strategy for stabilization, contributes to abdominal distension. Generally increased erythema (flushing) of their face and an inability to communicate because they are overly braced and bearing down will be noted. To combat this, use any of the previous suggestions above to help in controlling the issue, especially cuing them into their breathing.

a. Cue the individual's awareness of their transversus abdominis or pelvic floor by demonstrating where it is. Show them on a model or in a picture how the transversus abdominis wraps around the core, the pelvic floor covers the bottom of their pelvis, and how it is an analogous structure to the respiratory diaphragm.

b. Try any of the previous cues for activating the DMS and see which one resonates best with your client.

Maintaining the visualization, have the individual repeat their leg lift to see if it improves the quality of the movement. If none of these suggestions help with their control, it might be that the level of this pattern is too high for the individual to perform properly; in this case, choose the Pull-over pattern described below.

3. *Overuse of the superficial hip flexors.* Because of poor coordination between the deep and superficial myofascial systems, many individuals do not have a good strategy for lifting their leg, and will therefore overuse their superficial hip flexors. This may result in increased tension, tightness, and even cramping in their superficial hip flexors during hip flexion; this is a common contributor to femoroacetabular impingement syndrome (see Appendix V). To improve psoas activation and balance between the two myofascial systems, try the following:

a. Palpate, and/or have the individual palpate, their superficial hip flexors—the rectus femoris and tensor fasciae latae—and have them visualize drawing their leg up using the wire connection while cuing them to "soften" or "let go" with the superficial muscles. They should be able to initiate hip flexion prior to contraction of the superficial muscles.

b. Use the previous psoas, transversus abdominis and/or pelvic floor cues and have them repeat their hip flexion.

c. Foam roll and/or release around the hips to release restrictions, and repeat using the previous cues.

Heel Drop

Once the individual demonstrates proficiency in the Happy Baby position (they must be able to maintain their legs in the Happy Baby position for at least 3 sets of 3–5 breaths per set without compensations), they can be progressed to the Heel Drop. The Heel Drop pattern increases the psoas' role in both TPC stabilization and control during flexion and extension of the hip. Again, be sure the individual maintains TPC and hip alignment with three-dimensional breathing throughout the pattern.

Setting Up the Heel Drop Pattern

- The individual begins by lying supine, with their legs supported on a stability ball, coffee table, or chair, or with their feet flat upon the wall. They should be positioned as close to neutral as possible. From here they lift one leg at a time and hold their legs in the flexed position—this should be similar to the movement previously described in the Happy Baby position.

- From this position, they lower one leg at a time until their heel touches the surface, and then return their leg to the starting position (image top left overleaf). They then lower their other leg and return it to the starting position. As described earlier, there should be no change in the alignment of the spine, pelvis, or hips throughout the pattern.

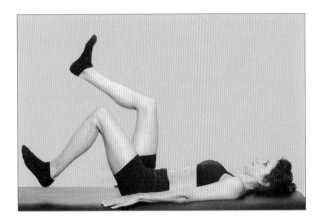

- The individual repeats the exercise for as long as they are able to maintain neutral alignment of their TPC and three-dimensional breathing. Be sure to monitor for the same compensations as noted earlier in the Happy Baby pattern.

For demonstration of the Heel Drop pattern, visit www.IIHFE.com/the-psoas-solution.

Pull-over

Although the psoas does not contribute to shoulder motion per se, as with the previous patterns it stabilizes the TPC against motion of the arms and against any external loads. Because of the benefits for core and shoulder stabilization, virtually every client and patient performs the Happy Baby with Pull-over pattern.

Benefits of the Pull-over pattern include:

- Many of the benefits of the Happy Baby pattern are also achieved—TPC stabilization and three-dimensional breathing with limb movement—without actually lifting the legs.
- The psoas and DMS control of neutral TPC alignment are trained with overhead motions of the arms—this is essential for developing control in overhead movements during everyday life, exercise, and sport.
- Eccentric lengthening of the latissimus dorsi is trained with a stable core—too frequently, the latissimus dorsi is trained without respecting TPC alignment.

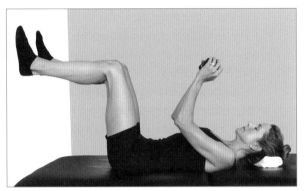

Setting Up the Pull-over Pattern

- The individual begins by lying supine, with their legs supported on a coffee table or chair, or with their feet flat upon the wall. They should be positioned as close to neutral as possible. Recall that the pelvis is in a slight anterior pelvic tilt, and that the curves of the spine are maintained (cervical and lumbar spines are lordotic, and the thorax is aligned with the pelvis). Motion of the arms should not cause any changes in the TPC alignment.
- The individual grasps a Pilates ring, yoga block, or light dumbbell, and holds it above their chest. Individuals who can raise their legs will use the previously described strategy; those who cannot lift their legs without losing control and maintaining their breathing can leave their legs in the supported position.

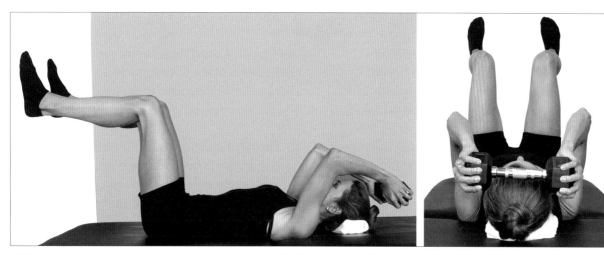

DB Pullovers in Happy Baby Supported Position—TPC alignment should be maintained throughout the pattern.

- The individual takes a breath in, and upon exhalation raises their arms overhead (image above left). TPC alignment should be maintained throughout the motion of their arms, without any gripping of the abdominal wall. The arms are brought back to the starting position during the next inhalation. The breathing pattern should consist of approximately 4 seconds for the eccentric phase (lengthening the arms overhead, and 2 seconds for returning the arms to the starting position (concentric phase). The elbows should remain equidistant apart from each other throughout the pattern (image above right).

For demonstration of the Pull-over pattern, visit www.IIHFE.com/the-psoas-solution.

Common Signs of Dysfunction in the Pull-over

Similar compensations to those discussed earlier in the Happy Baby pattern may occur during the Pull-over pattern. The issue that most commonly presents is excessive rib cage flare, associated with thoracolumbar extension as the arms are brought into the overhead position. This generally occurs for one of the following three reasons and is usually corrected quite easily using an appropriate strategy:

1. The control required to stabilize the TPC with overhead motion has not been developed (or control is compromised during the pattern). These individuals need to be taught, or reminded, how to breathe and to activate the

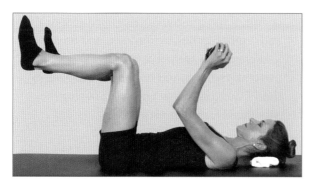
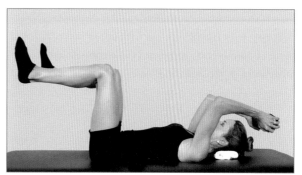

DB Pullovers in Happy Baby Unsupported Position—The individual should be able to maintain alignment, breathing, and TPC control throughout the pattern.

DMS, before being reintroduced to the Pull-over pattern.

2. The individual does not have adequate latissimus dorsi length. Manual release, foam rolling, or gentle stretching with TPC alignment can help to improve latissimus dorsi length. Repeat the pattern after the latissimus dorsi has been released, and note if the individual is then able to maintain TPC alignment.

3. Too much resistance and/or too great a range of motion is being used. Lower the resistance and/or shorten the range of motion, and note whether the individual can then maintain more optimal TPC alignment.

Pull-over with Heel Drop

Once the individual demonstrates proficiency in both the Happy Baby and Pull-over patterns, they can be progressed to the Pull-over with Heel Drop. Again, be sure that the individual maintains TPC alignment with three-dimensional breathing during the movement of the extremities.

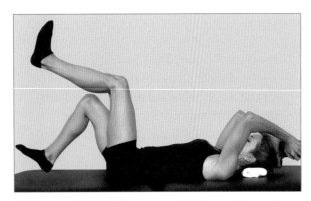

Pull-over with Heel Drop—as with the previous patterns there should be no change in TPC alignment with movement of the arms and legs.

Modified Dead Bug

The Modified Dead Bug is aptly named, as it is a modification of the traditional Dead Bug pattern. There are several benefits of the Modified Dead Bug pattern over the traditional version:

1. For most individuals the Modified Dead Bug makes it easier to focus on TPC control and movement of the legs, compared with trying to control the TPC in the traditional version of the exercise with all four limbs moving.

2. Because of the gentle pressing action into a wall, the Modified Dead Bug pattern generally makes it easier to engage the core muscles and control TPC alignment. Pressing into the wall also makes it easier to stabilize the TLJ and activate the psoas in the control of hip motion.

3. With gentle pressing into the wall, the Modified Dead Bug pattern coordinates the control of overhead motion with TPC alignment and three-dimensional breathing.

Setting Up the Modified Dead Bug Pattern

• The individual begins by lying supine, with their legs in the hook lying position and with their head near a wall. They should be positioned as close to neutral as possible. Recall that neutral alignment is where the pelvis is in a slight anterior pelvic tilt, and the curves of the spine are maintained (cervical and lumbar spines are lordotic, and the thorax is aligned with the pelvis). As in the previous patterns, there should not be any changes in the TPC alignment at any point during the Modified Dead Bug pattern.

- The individual takes a few three-dimensional breaths; upon inhaling, they lift their arms so that their palms are flat on the wall (image below). They lightly engage, or push into, the wall and take a few more breaths before resting and repeating.

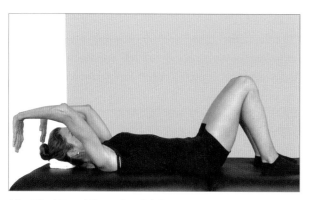

Modified Dead Bug—hook lying.

- Similar to the Happy Baby progression, they can begin coordinating leg lifting. They should begin by lifting one leg on an inhalation, return it to the surface on the corresponding exhalation, and then repeat this procedure with the other leg.
- If the individual has demonstrated optimal alignment and control, they can progress to lifting both legs, and perform 1–5 breaths with the legs elevated (image right). Make sure that they control their TPC alignment and breathing while both maintaining their legs elevated as well as when lifting and lowering their legs.

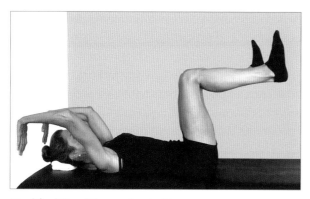

Modified Dead Bug—elevated legs.

- The pattern can be progressed by performing the heel drop and/or moving further away from the wall. Ensure the individual maintains TPC alignment and breathing throughout the pattern.

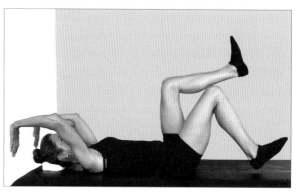

Modified Dead Bug—heel drops.

For demonstration of the Modified Dead Bug pattern, visit www.IIHFE.com/the-psoas-solution.

Common Signs of Dysfunction in the Modified Dead Bug

During the Modified Dead Bug similar compensations to those seen in the Happy Baby and Pull-over patterns may occur—thoracolumbar extension, posterior pelvic tilt and lumbar spine flexion, and an inability to maintain three-dimensional breathing. Use the same correction strategies mentioned in the other patterns in order to correct any alterations in alignment, breathing, or control throughout the pattern.

Clinical Consideration: Abdominal Hollowing Versus Bracing Stabilization Strategies

There has been an ongoing debate about which core activation strategy—abdominal hollowing (AH) or bracing—is the best for stabilizing the spine. The Queensland group of Hodges and colleagues has been associated with AH as a core activation strategy in the presence of timing delays and faulty recruitment of the transversus abdominis in individuals experiencing low back pain. On the other hand, McGill (2007) has advocated an approach that favors bracing or co-activation of the core muscles to stiffen and stabilize the spine. McGill's research demonstrates that abdominal hollowing, or drawing the abdominals in, reduces spinal stability.

After studying with Hodges, as well as with several individuals that share similar strategies with the Queensland group, including renowned physical therapists Diane Lee and Dr. Linda-Joy Lee (who completed her Ph.D. at the University of Queensland) it has not been suggested that, to stabilize the spine or solve one's back problems, all one needs to do is hollow or activate the transversus abdominis. It appears this thinking likely stems from individuals who have interpreted the research and have chosen to focus solely upon one aspect alone (i.e. the need for AH), and have discounted the bigger clinical picture of the research. In fact, research conclusively and consistently demonstrates that individuals with chronic pain demonstrate timing delays and often atrophy of the deeper, intrinsic muscles, compared with individuals not experiencing pain. Moreover, the research supports that often individuals experiencing chronic pain benefit from specific training focused on activating the deeper, intrinsic muscles (including the transversus abdominis, multifidi, pelvic floor, and psoas) to restore function and decrease pain.

Where does this seemingly conflicting information leave the trainer, clinician or therapist who work with individuals who are experiencing chronic low back pain or, for that matter, hip and pelvic dysfunction?

Clinicians, therapists, and fitness professionals, are often left having to decide which approach one favors and feel is most "right." Rather than taking an "either or" approach to deciding which core stabilization strategy one favors, an "and" should be included in the equation. In other words, there are situations when one should be specific and teach the motor control strategies favored by Hodges and his co-workers at the Queensland group, Dr. Linda-Joy Lee, Diane Lee, Sean Gibbons, and others, *and* there are situations when bracing strategies—i.e. the McGill approach—are more appropriate. The challenge comes in knowing when and with whom to use the appropriate strategy.

As discussed in this chapter, inhibition of the DMS can be a contributor to, and/or the result of, chronic pain. Bracing strategies, which are inherently more effective in activating the SMS than the DMS, have not clinically demonstrated effectiveness in rectifying atrophy of the DMS or in decreasing overactivity of the SMS—two common indicators of a non-optimal core stabilization strategy.

In conclusion, both approaches—AH and bracing—have their respective places in a well-designed rehabilitation and/or training program. Experience and expertise, as well as client population, will dictate which approach to use and when best to apply it. Many individuals who have chronic pain, chronic tightness, and/or the loss of performance will require a strategy that encourages the use of *both* strategies.

Modified Wall Plank

The Modified Wall Plank pattern was initially developed with the goal of improving an individual's scapular stabilization while in the upright position; it has turned out to be a great pattern for training optimal posture and alignment. The Modified Wall Plank is also beneficial for those individuals who struggle to achieve optimal TPC alignment when face down, as well as those who cannot tolerate the prone position. It is also useful for training optimal alignment and control of the head, neck, shoulder complex, and TPC in the upright position. Additionally, the Modified Wall Plank is one of the more effective patterns for developing optimal postural awareness, and can easily be performed anywhere there is a wall or a door. It is a prerequisite for the hip flexion progression that will be discussed below.

Setting Up the Modified Wall Plank Pattern

- The individual aligns and stacks their TPC (they should be in neutral alignment) and then places her forearms flat against the wall, as in the prone position for the Prone Lengthen (images below). Her hands start at chin level,

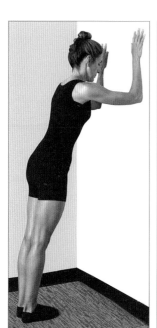 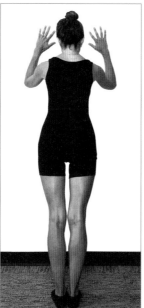

with her thumbs pointing toward each other. Next, she'll take a small step away from the wall; she should be leaning slightly into the wall at this point.
- Cue the individual: "Stay open and wide through the front of your shoulders, and lengthen through the back of your head as if you are being gently pulled toward the ceiling." In this position they take 3–5 three-dimensional breaths, focusing on filling up their TPC.
- After the individual has taken the last of the breaths, they extend their arms and push themselves off the wall, dropping their arms to their sides. If they have performed the pattern well, this will be their most neutral TPC alignment. As mentioned previously, this is an excellent pattern in which to train postural awareness and control, as well as providing a great postural mini-break for office workers and for those individuals in repetitive occupations.

Modified Wall Plank with Hip Flexion

The Modified Wall Plank with Hip Flexion is a great pattern to incorporate the psoas into upright function. There are several benefits of the Modified Wall Plank with Hip Flexion:

1. It teaches optimal alignment of the TPC, scapula, head, and neck in a modified plank type of position.
2. By pressing lightly into a wall, the individual will find that the Modified Wall Plank pattern generally makes it easier to engage the core muscles and control TPC alignment. Pressing into the wall also makes it easier to stabilize the TLJ and activate the psoas in the control of hip motion.
3. The slightly inclined position of the body is an easier method for teaching optimal hip flexion than the upright position.

4. It is an effective pattern for improving gluteal activation and lengthening of the superficial hip flexors on the stationary or stance leg.

5. It is a great way to teach posture and balance, and to begin gait training in a very safe exercise position, even for older adults.

Setting Up the Modified Wall Plank with Hip Flexion

- The individual begins in the Modified Wall Plank position: their forearms are against the wall so that their thumbs are about level with their ears (image below left). They visualize being long from the back of their head, and feel as if they are gently pulling the wall apart between their hands.

- They begin by lifting one leg on an inhalation (image below right), return it to the floor on the corresponding exhalation, and then repeat this procedure with the other leg. Flexion of the hip should not cause any change to neutral alignment of the TPC. A good cue is to encourage the individual to lift their knee toward the wall without moving their pelvis. (Note: it may be necessary to cue the individual as to when their pelvis moves, as many individuals will not be aware of this motion.)

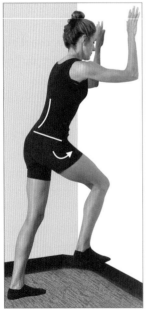

For demonstration of the Modified Wall Plank with Hip Extension pattern, visit www.IIHFE.com/the-psoas-solution.

Common Signs of Dysfunction in the Modified Wall Plank with Hip Flexion

There are two common dysfunctions that can manifest during this pattern:

1. *Lifting the leg too high.* This encourages the pelvis to move into posterior rotation and the lumbar spine to flex (image below). The individual should be cued to maintain neutral alignment, and to stop lifting their leg just prior to the point where they are losing neutral alignment.

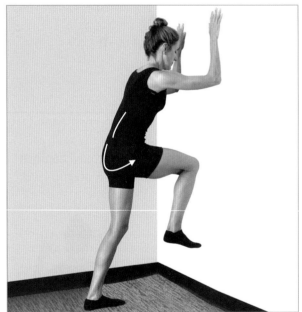

Modified Wall Plank with Hip Flexion—commonly, individuals will lift their leg beyond their range of hip flexion resulting in posterior pelvic rotation and lumbar spine flexion. This is a common compensation which results in perpetuation of non-optimal alignment and control of the TPC and hip.

2. *Loss of spinal and/or pelvic.* This often occurs when the individual has lost core control (usually at the TLJ), has a non-optimal breathing strategy, and/or has a poor dissociation strategy for hip flexion which causes the spine or pelvis to shift (image below).

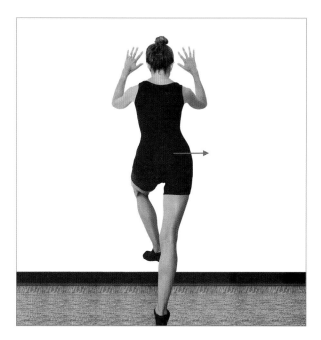

a. To improve TLJ stability, cue them to take a deep breath and elongate just before lifting their leg.
b. If their breathing seems to be compromised, begin with the Happy Baby or Modified Dead Bug pattern to teach proper breathing and TLJ stability prior to attempting the Modified Wall Plank pattern.
c. If they have poor hip dissociation, perform myofascial release on the structures around the hip, before repeating this pattern using the cues from the earlier Happy Baby and Modified Dead Bug patterns.

Once the individual can perform 8–10 repetitions with no compensations, they can be progressed to an inclined surface. The Bench Plank with Hip Flexion pattern is an excellent higher-level pattern for developing core stabilization with hip

flexion, while incorporating postural alignment and control. Ensure that the individual maintains neutral alignment during the hip flexion phase of the pattern especially as they transition between sides.

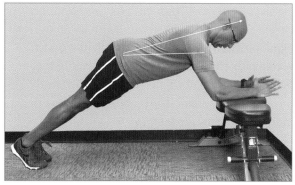

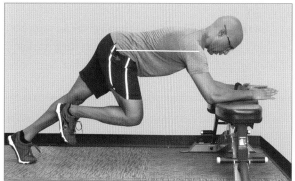

Bench Plank with Hip Flexion—The individual should maintain neutral TPC alignment with hip flexion.

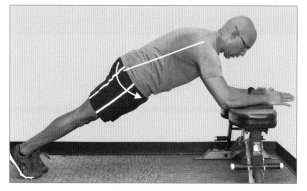

It is common for individuals to compromise their TPC alignment because of limited hip flexion range of motion and/or by overusing their abdominal wall, which flexes the spine and pulls the pelvis into posterior tilt (image above).

Ball-supported Knee Pull-in

The Ball-supported Knee Pull-in pattern is a high-level core stabilization exercise that incorporates the psoas and superficial hip flexors. Ball-supported Knee Pull-ins are essentially a plank pattern performed with hip flexion; therefore ensure that the individual can maintain an optimal plank position and is able to execute the Bench Plank with Hip Flexion before performing the Ball-supported Knee Pull-in pattern. Generally it is best to use a ball that is about as wide as the individual's arms are long.

Setting Up the Ball-supported Knee Pull-in Pattern

- The individual positions themselves in neutral TPC alignment over the ball, with their tibias or feet placed over the ball (image below).

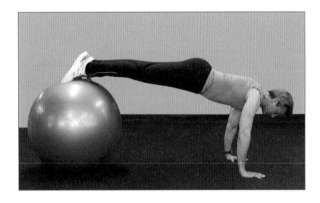

- The individual flexes their hips and knees while maintaining neutral alignment. They should visualize keeping their tailbone pointed up and behind them, and their knees should be pointed toward the floor rather than towards their chest (image above right). They pull their knees in as far as they can without losing neutral alignment of their TPC.

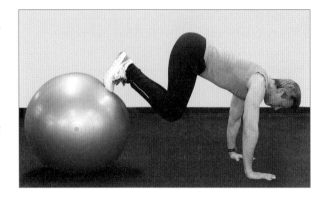

- Maintaining neutral alignment, they extend their hips to return to the starting position.
- The individual maintains TPC alignment as they flex and extend their hips.

Common Signs of Dysfunction in the Ball-supported Knee Pull-in

Several common compensations can occur with the Ball-supported Knee Pull-in pattern:

1. *Not maintaining TPC alignment.* It is common for many individuals performing this pattern to lose neutral TPC alignment, especially as they fatigue. Have them stop, and give them a break. If they cannot maintain neutral alignment throughout the pattern, regress them to a static plank pattern and/or the inclined hip flexion pattern described earlier.
2. *Pulling into posterior pelvic tilt and lumbar spine flexion.* This is related to point 1 above. For many individuals the level of this pattern is too great, and they will compensate by posteriorly tilting and flexing their lumbar spine in an attempt to stabilize their TPC. Cue them into more optimal alignment, and if they are still unable to remain in this position, regress them to a more appropriate pattern in which they are able to maintain neutral alignment.
3. *Loss of scapular control.* Generally, if the individual loses scapular control, this is not the best pattern for them. If they cannot be easily cued into more optimal scapular alignment, regress them to a pattern in which they are able to maintain control.

Summary of Psoas Function in Happy Baby, Pull-over, Modified Dead Bug, Modified Wall Plank with Hip Flexion, Bench Plank with Hip Flexion, and Ball-supported Knee Pull-in Patterns

Psoas function at the trunk, spine, and pelvis
- Stabilizes the TLJ, lumbar spine, and pelvis to assist in maintaining TPC alignment and three-dimensional breathing during leg or arm movement.

Psoas function at the hip
- Centrates the femoral head within the acetabulum during hip flexion.
- From a flexed position, the psoas functions eccentrically to control the hip as the leg is extending.

Summary: Core Stabilization Patterns

1. During core stabilization patterns (and their variations), the psoas functions as a stabilizer of the spine and pelvis, so that the TPC remains in neutral alignment. In particular, the psoas stabilizes and anchors the TLJ, lumbar spine, and pelvis to help maintain integrity of the TPC.

2. The psoas axially compresses (stiffens) the lumbar spine, which helps maintain lumbar lordosis during hip flexion and extension.

3. The psoas works with the lower fibers of the gluteus maximus to maintain femoral head centration within the acetabulum during both flexion and extension of the hip. This enables the hips to remain centrated, which directly contributes to the ability to maintain the pelvis in a neutral (anterior pelvic tilt) and level position throughout the core exercise patterns.

Signs of non-optimal psoas function during core exercise patterns:
- Loss of lumbar lordosis (flexion of the spine) when flexing the hip especially in lower ranges.
- Lack of posterior glide of the femoral head, resulting in early and/or excessive spinal flexion and posterior pelvic rotation during hip flexion.
- Excessive extension at the TLJ during core exercise patterns.
- Excessive anterior translation of the femoral head during hip extension (returning to the starting position from a hip-flexed position).
- Unleveling (frontal plane motion) and/or rotation (transverse plane motion) of the pelvis during any point of the pattern.

Squat and Deadlifting

- Importance and benefits of the squatting and deadlifting patterns in life and sport
- Psoas' role in spinal and pelvic stabilization as well as in hip centration during the squatting and deadlifting patterns
- Optimal performance of the squatting and deadlifting patterns and how to identify common signs of loss of control related to the psoas

Introduction

The Squat and Deadlift (traditional form) patterns are two of the fundamental patterns for life. Both squatting and deadlifting provide the ability to lower one's center of mass toward the ground and either hold oneself in this position or safely and efficiently lift heavy objects from the ground. For most individuals, squatting is one of the safest methods for working on the ground without placing increased stress upon the spine and pelvis.

While it cannot be argued that the prolonged seated posture has a high likelihood of leading to

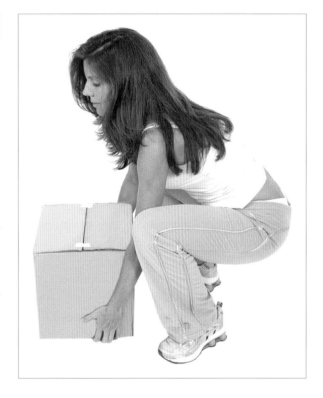

musculoskeletal and soft tissues problems, there are many problems associated with sitting, which have more to do with not being able to achieve optimal pelvic and hip alignment than with the act of sitting itself. The ability to sit properly with support upon the ischial tuberosities (sits bones) and align the thoracopelvic cylinder (TPC)

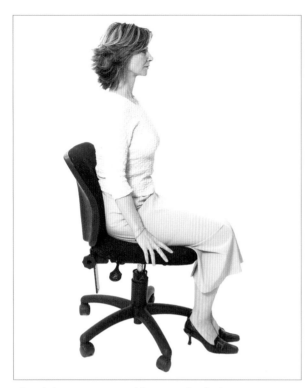

The ability to squat enables an individual to sit upon their ischial tuberosities (sits bones) and properly align their trunk and spine over their pelvis.

over the pelvis stems from the squat. Sitting is therefore essentially a supported squat position. See addendum for more on adopting an ideal sitting posture.

There are many benefits to being able to optimally squat and deadlift, including:

- Squatting and deadlifting train alignment and control of the trunk, spine, and pelvis as well as the lower extremities in the upright position.
- Squatting and deadlifting are two of the most efficient ways of lifting heavy objects from the ground and/or positioning oneself to work at ground level.
- Optimally loading the hips during a squat or deadlift pattern mobilizes the soft tissue and lubricates the hip joints (stimulates production and release of synovial fluid).
- Squatting grooves the hip and TPC alignment required for optimal sitting.
- Optimal alignment while squatting and deadlifting prevents excessive pressure on the

low back caused by the inability to properly align the trunk, spine, and/or pelvis.
- When loaded with weights—barbells, dumbbells, kettlebells, etc.—squatting and deadlifting patterns are excellent exercises for conditioning the core (the TPC) and entire lower extremity.
- When performed in a fast manner, or in combination with overhead presses, chops, and other exercise patterns, squatting becomes an excellent tool for metabolic conditioning.

Psoas' Role in Squatting and Deadlifting

There are three primary ways in which the psoas contributes to optimal squatting and deadlifting:

1. The psoas helps stabilize and maintain lumbar lordosis through the early to mid phases of the squatting and deadlifting patterns, and prevents excessive spinal flexion (flattening of the lumbar spine) in the mid to late phases of the squat.
2. The psoas helps to maintain a neutral pelvis position (anterior pelvic rotation) in the early to mid phases of the squatting and deadlifting patterns; this additionally helps to maintain lumbar lordosis and overall alignment of the TPC.
3. The psoas and lower glutes help centrate the femoral head within the acetabulum. Together, these muscles ensure optimal hip flexion (hip hinge) and maintenance of neutral pelvic and spinal alignment during the early to mid phases of the squatting or deadlifting patterns. In the later phase of the squatting pattern, optimal hip centration keeps the pelvis from moving excessively into posterior rotation.

Breathing Strategy During the Squatting and Deadlifting Patterns

Breathing is critical to optimal performance during the squatting and deadlifting patterns. There are three general breathing strategies that can be used in the various squatting and deadlifting patterns discussed in this chapter:

1. *When performing bodyweight Squats or Deadlifts and the goal is to groove the pattern.* The individual inhales prior to the start of the repetition, exhales as they lower into the squat, and inhales as they rise out of it. Clinically this breathing strategy helps to coordinate activity between the diaphragm and pelvic floor and release myofascial gripping around the hip joint to restore more optimal hip motion.
2. *When using light to moderate external loads in the Squat and Deadlift patterns.* The repetitions are generally performed in cadence with the individual's breathing: the individual inhales as they lower into the Squat or Deadlift pattern, and exhales as they rise out of it. This is the traditional pattern of breathing used during resistance training.
3. *When using higher to near-maximum loads in the squat and deadlift patterns.* The goal with breathing during heavier training is to maximize intra-abdominal and intra-thoracic pressures (pressures within the thoracopelvic cylinder) to maintain trunk, spine, and pelvic stability. Therefore, the individual takes a deep breath in and holds it during the eccentric (lowering) phase, then slowly exhales (maintaining relative internal pressure) during the concentric phase; they only fully exhale once they have reached the lockout phase at the end of the motion.

Inhaling and holding one's breath has been shown to develop greater intra-abdominal pressure (Hagins et al. 2004) and may be beneficial for well-trained individuals who are performing heavy lifting. A more important consideration than exactly how the individual is breathing is that the individual maintains a breathing strategy appropriate to the intensity of current exercise and that they are not holding their breath. See the breathing chapter (Chapter 2) for more specifics regarding breathing and exercise.

Improving Hip Extension During Squatting and Deadlifting Patterns

Naturally, every lower extremity pattern has a flexion as well as an extension phase to it. This section will briefly discuss the mechanics involved in the *hip extension* phases of the Squat and Deadlift patterns discussed in this book, as well as of the Lunge pattern (which will be covered in Chapter 5), since the mechanics for these patterns are quite similar.

In an attempt to counteract the impact of the *lower crossed syndrome*—excessive anterior pelvic tilt and lumbar hyperlordosis—many individuals who go through rehabilitation and/or training programs are being trained into excessive hip extension. Cues to over-activate the gluteus maximus at the end of squat, deadlift, lunge, and other lower extremity exercise patterns are commonplace in both rehabilitation and training environments.

An unfortunate consequence of this cuing strategy is that increasing numbers of individuals are demonstrating a condition clinically referred to as *extension syndrome*. In extension syndrome the individual presents with overly contracted and developed spinal and hip extensors, which generally leads to excessive thoracic spine extension, posterior pelvic tilt, and hip extension in quiet standing (Osar 2012, 2015). As a result, they will tend to be positioned in lumbar spine flexion, and have *anterior femoral glide syndrome*, in which their femoral heads have translated excessively anteriorly and are over-compressed within the acetabulum. These postural changes—which will ultimately impact movement quality, as will be discussed in the dysfunction section below—inhibit the individual's ability to optimally use both the psoas and the deep gluteus maximus fibers in joint centration, thus affecting hip function during activities of daily living and exercise.

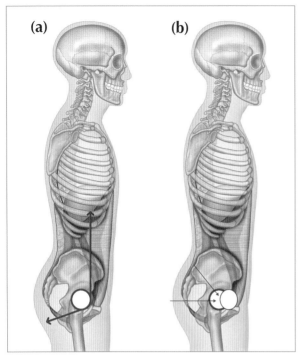

The psoas and lower fibers of the gluteus maximus work synergistically to maintain hip centration, alignment, and control of the femoral head during the squat and deadlift patterns. The arrows in the image above indicate the relative direction of pull of the psoas (superior) and lower gluteus maximus fibers (posterior) in maintaining hip centration (a). With over-contraction of the superficial fibers of gluteus maximus and posterior fibers of gluteus medius, the pelvis is pulled into posterior pelvic rotation and the femoral head is driven forward within the acetabulum (b).

One of the most effective strategies for simultaneously improving gluteus maximus and psoas function is to ensure that the individual has optimal TPC alignment at the beginning of their exercise pattern, and to cue them appropriately at the end of the pattern.

Improving Psoas and Gluteal Function During Squatting and Deadlifting Patterns

- Ensure that the individual is initially set up properly:

  - neutral TPC (thorax stacked and suspended over the pelvis) and hip alignment
  - head and neck alignment over the TPC
  - lower extremity alignment (foot tripod, and the hip, knee, ankle-foot complex in a relatively straight line)
- During the eccentric (lowering) phase, the individual focuses on releasing through the posterior hip, and/or softening through the anterior hip, as they sit back into their hips. This concept of releasing or 'sitting back in the hips' should be developed with bodyweight prior to loading.
- During the concentric (rising) phase, cue the individual to drive the top or crown of their head up toward the ceiling to return to the starting position. Avoid cuing them to "squeeze" or "contract" their glutes, or to "drive the pelvis forward," as they return to the starting position.

If they have maintained TPC alignment throughout the pattern, they will have to use their glutes to lift themselves out of the bottom position of the exercise, and these muscles will remain active throughout the pattern. Therefore, the individual should not have to be cued to activate their glutes.

Squat

The discussion that follows will focus on maintaining neutral alignment of the TPC (thorax stacked over the pelvis, lumbar lordosis, and anterior pelvic rotation) throughout the squatting pattern. The individual will therefore only be squatting to a depth that allows them to maintain neutral alignment. A discussion of deep, or end-range, squatting will be included at the end of this section.

Clinical Consideration: Reciprocal Inhibition of the Psoas

The concept of reciprocal inhibition has been a staple of rehabilitation and corrective exercise approaches for the past few decades. In an attempt to counter the dreaded anterior pelvic tilt and increased lumbar lordosis syndrome, and to lengthen its culprit—the short, tight, and overactive psoas—many health and fitness professionals will cue their clients or patients to "squeeze" their glutes at the end of the hip extension patterns.

The basis of this approach is Sherrington's Law of Reciprocal Inhibition, which suggests that the contraction of a muscle will inhibit its antagonist. This strategy has led to an array of industry cues focused on activating the glutes in order to inhibit their antagonist, the psoas. These cues include (but are not limited to): "Squeeze your cheeks as hard as you can," "Squeeze your cheeks as if you have a million dollars between them," and "Tuck your pelvis and tighten your tush." Unfortunately, these approaches often fail to improve gluteal function during functional tasks or exercises.

Since the psoas rarely is the lone culprit leading to an increased lumbar lordosis, and anatomically cannot cause an anterior pelvic tilt (review functional anatomy in Chapter 1), there are three problems with the above concept and use of the Law of Reciprocal Inhibition:

1. It assumes that contraction of the glutes inhibits and therefore prevents the individual from contracting their superficial hip flexors. Clinically, it is commonplace that individuals merely develop excessive co-contraction of both their superficial glutes and their hip flexors. This strategy ultimately leads to greater compression of the hips.
2. Practitioners and trainers using the above cues are not ensuring that the femoral heads remain centrated within the acetabula. Many individuals are over-contracting their glutes (as well as their deep hip rotators) and causing their femoral heads to be driven forward within the acetabula. Over-activation of the superficial gluteus maximus tends to inhibit the use of the deeper gluteal fibers as well as of the psoas. This further perpetuates the anterior femoral head position and overall dysfunctional gluteal activity.
3. Over-contracting the glutes pulls the pelvis into a posterior pelvic tilt, which consequently flattens the lumbar spine. This will further inhibit gluteal and psoas function, and subsequently increase stress both on the lumbar spine and on the sacroiliac joints.

These results are undesirable and will dramatically impact psoas function, and therefore optimal control of the spine, pelvis, and hips. This approach contributes to femoroacetabular impingement (FAI), sacroiliac joint issues, and lumbar disc problems.

To promote optimal co-activation of the gluteus maximus and psoas, educate the patient or client in how to use their hips appropriately. Should there be a need to have them actively focus on contracting their glutes, then ensure that their hips remain centrated and that their pelvis remains neutrally positioned.

To educate individuals to optimally use their glutes without over-activating them, a helpful cue is: "Use, don't crush, your glutes." Teach the individual how to align and control neutral alignment of their TPC and hips, and how to integrate use of their psoas and DMS; more often than not, their glute function will improve accordingly.

Setting Up the Squat Pattern

- The individual starts with their feet about shoulder-width apart. The feet should be supported like a tripod, meaning that most of the pressure will be under the first metatarsophalangeal joint (or big-toe side of the foot), the fifth metatarsophalangeal joint (or little-toe side of the foot), and the calcaneus (heel). The hip, knee, ankle, and foot should be aligned with each other so that a straight line goes from the hip joint, through the inside to middle of the knee joint, and to a point between the first and second digits of the foot (image left).

- The individual aligns their trunk over their pelvis—essentially they are stacking their TPC. They should be in a relatively neutral spinal alignment, and the lower opening of the rib cage should face toward their feet and not forward. The pelvis should be neutrally aligned (anterior pelvic tilt), with their anterior superior iliac

spines (ASISs) slightly anterior to (in front of) their pubic symphysis. An ability to achieve this alignment is a good indication that the psoas is functioning properly.

- The first movement in the Squat pattern should be a hip hinge, or flexion of the hips, which translates the pelvis posteriorly however the pelvis remains in an anteriorly rotated position (image below right). This movement will in turn lead to knee flexion and ankle dorsiflexion. As the individual lowers their body, they should be able to keep their TPC stacked and their pelvis relatively neutral until all their available hip flexion is used up. To ensure a safe squatting position for the spine and pelvis, the individual only squats within the range through which they are able to maintain neutral pelvic alignment, and therefore neutral spinal alignment. It is important to note that full-range squatting will require a posterior pelvic tilt and slight lumbar flexion; however, the initial goal is to

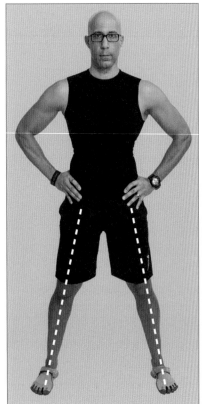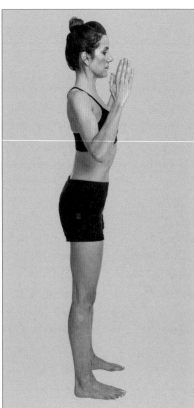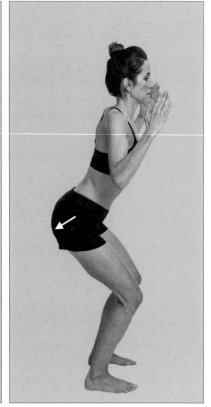

Squat Pattern—front view (left); side view (middle); initiation of the squat (right)—the individual flexes (hinges) their hips and sits back (arrow).

teach individuals to control neutral alignment, and master the Squat pattern with neutral alignment before they learn to move out of this position. See more on this in the discussion of the deep, or end-range, squat.

- The individual lifts out of the bottom of the pattern to return to the starting position in exactly the same TPC alignment. They should be using (but not over-contracting) their glute complex (gluteus maximus, medius, and minimus) and hamstrings to rise from the bottom position.

While it is a common cue to instruct individuals to activate, or "squeeze," their glutes at the top of the Squat pattern, this will tend to posteriorly rotate the pelvis and/or drive the femoral head anteriorly within the acetabulum.

To facilitate more optimal movement of the hip joint, while ensuring co-activation of the psoas and glutes, there are several cues that are helpful:

- Individuals are encouraged to "sit back" with their hips (eccentrically lengthening the glutes) and cued to "spread," "lengthen," or "let go" during the lowering phase in order to ensure proper posterior glide of the femoral head within the acetabulum.
- Individuals are encouraged to lift their body up toward the ceiling (concentrically shortening the glutes), allowing their glutes to work, but without encouragement to over-activate and/or "squeeze" them at the end of the pattern. They should be cued to "lift the head toward the ceiling" to ensure that they are lifting their body up, rather than translating their pelvis forward. This glute strategy helps maintain optimal length and tension in the psoas.

For demonstration of the Squat pattern, visit www. IIHFE.com/the-psoas-solution.

Once the individual has mastered the basic squatting movement, appropriate loading can be added to the pattern. The front-loaded (or goblet) squat is preferred to back loading (with a barbell),

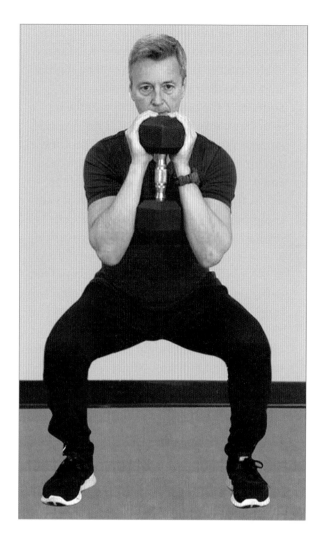

as it is the easiest way to load the pattern while respecting TPC alignment and control (image above). Ensure that the load does not compromise the individual's alignment, breathing, and control during the pattern.

Common Signs of Dysfunction in the Squat

There are three common signs that indicate non-optimal psoas involvement during the Squat pattern:

1. *Non-optimal TPC alignment at the beginning.* Many individuals begin their patterns in a posterior pelvic tilt and lumbar spine flexion position. The individual must often be taught the position of neutral pelvic alignment, and

how to maintain it during the Squat pattern. Have the individual palpate their ASIS and pubic symphysis: the ASIS should be slightly anterior to their pubic symphysis.

Stiffness in the posterior portion of the hip joint capsule, or in the posterior hip muscles (superficial glute max, hamstrings, piriformis), can limit posterior glide of the femoral head and contribute to posterior rotation of the pelvis. Restrictions in any of these areas can compromise optimal psoas function. Self-myofascial release, manual therapy release, and/or verbal or tactile cuing can be effective in helping the individual release and maintain optimal psoas function, and thereby maintain centration of the hips and a more ideal pelvic alignment.

Oftentimes, the individual must be instructed to suspend their thorax, which essentially lifts their thorax up and over the pelvis, allowing the pelvis to return to a more neutral alignment. Review the concept of rib cage suspension in Appendix III.

2. *Starting posterior pelvic tilt and lumbar spine flexion too early.* During an ideal Squat pattern, the pelvis should not posteriorly rotate until approximately 90–120° of hip flexion. This range will be determined by the individual's specific hip range of motion and will therefore vary from person to person. Early posterior tilt and lumbar spine flexion tends to inhibit the psoas, and indicates that the individual has posterior joint capsule restriction, posterior myofascial tension, and/or is not actively letting their hip muscles relax enough to ensure optimal hip centration.

Self-myofascial release, manual therapy release, and/or verbal or tactile cuing can be effective in helping the individual to release the areas they are holding and to maintain centration of the hips. Verbal cues, including "Sit your hips back," "Release from your posterior hips," "Let your sits bones go wide," and "Think of letting the ball sink back in the socket," can encourage more-ideal posterior femoral

head glide. Activation of the psoas and other muscles of the deep myofascial system (DMS) can additionally be effective in rebalancing the muscles around the hip and in reducing excessive levels of tone or gripping.

For those who are new to the Squat pattern, or have spent years over-activating the posterior hip complex, there may be a feeling that they are about to fall backward when they are actually releasing from their posterior hip complex. The Supported Squat pattern (see p. 102) should be performed to help individuals groove the motion, and provide them with the ability to focus on their alignment and on letting go without the fear of falling backward.

3. *Excessive extension at the thoracolumbar junction (TLJ).* Many individuals stand in a position of posterior pelvic rotation with lumbar spine flexion. They often compensate for this by hyperextending at the TLJ—the region where the lower thorax meets the upper lumbar spine. The issue is also common when the individual leans their trunk too far forward in the Squat pattern, and then compensates for this by extending at their TLJ. Hyperextension at the TLJ is especially problematic, as it will overstretch and inhibit the psoas and abdominal wall, which compromises alignment and control of the TPC and hence spinal stability.

To improve TPC alignment, cue the client to lower their thorax so that it is stacked on top of their pelvis. A simple way to kinesthetically cue them into a more ideal TPC alignment is to have them place their hands in one of three regions:

i. Their middle finger of one hand on their umbilicus (belly button) and their thumb on the xiphoid process.

ii. One hand on their chest and one on their lower abdomen (images opposite).

iii. Their middle fingers over their ASISs, and their thumbs on their lower rib cage (if their fingers are long enough).

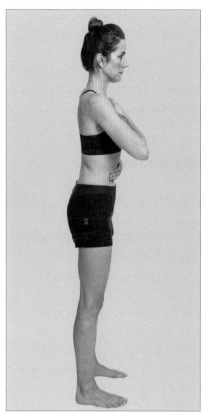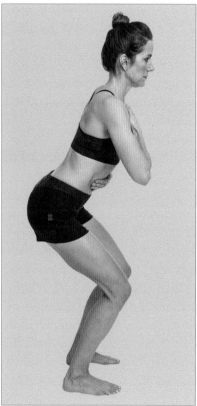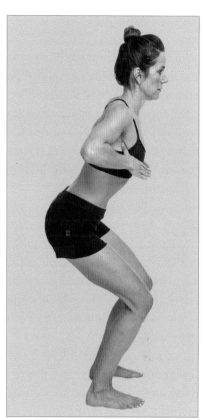

Monitoring TPC alignment—placing hands on chest and abdomen (left and middle images); placing hands on upper rib cage to enhance suspension (image right).

The goal is to maintain the distance between their hands or fingers throughout the pattern; if their fingers or hands separate during the pattern, they are likely overextending at the TLJ.

Cuing suspension of the thorax is also an extremely effective strategy for maintaining TPC alignment and three-dimensional breathing during the Squat pattern. The individual places their hands on either sides of their rib cage (image above right); they visualize gently wrapping their ribs back toward the spine, and keeping the back of their rib cage suspended toward the ceiling throughout the Squat pattern.

Clinical Consideration

Over-activation of the posterior hip complex, and the resultant posterior pelvic tilt and lumbar spine flexion, will cause and perpetuate psoas inhibition. It is important to teach psoas activation and ensure that the patient controls neutral alignment of the pelvis (slight anterior pelvic tilt) prior to moving them out of this position. For individuals experiencing chronic low back and/or hip irritation, it is most beneficial to keep them moving through shorter ranges in the squat pattern, rather than moving them through deeper ranges where they cannot optimally control spine, pelvis, and/or hip alignment.

Supported Squat

While it can technically be viewed as a regression, the Supported Squat is an ideal pattern for educating an individual about how to maintain TPC alignment while releasing myofascial tension through their hips. This allows the individual to focus on their technique of releasing and sitting back in their hips without the fear of falling backward.

Nearly every patient who clinically presents with low back, hip, and lower extremity dysfunction will perform the Supported Squat pattern as part of their corrective exercise strategy. For clients in general training, the Supported Squat is usually programmed as part of their functional warm-up.

The individual can grasp a machine, the doorknobs of an open door, or suspension straps, and/or simply place their hands on the wall for support (images below). While the mechanics and cues from the Squat above are incorporated into the supported version, there will be a difference in how the individual breathes during the pattern. To facilitate eccentric release of the glutes and posterior hip complex, the individual will breathe in as they ascend, and they will breathe out and relax the hips fully as they descend into the pattern.

For demonstration of the Supported Squat pattern, visit www.IIHFE.com/the-psoas-solution.

Deep, or End-range, Squat

In any conversation about squatting, the question invariably arises as to how deep one should squat. Proponents of deep, or end-range, squatting (squatting to the point where the posterior hips meet the back of the lower legs) will, in support of their way of thinking, point to examples of babies, cavemen, and individuals in cultures where deep squatting is performed throughout their entire lives (e.g. in Asia, Africa, and India).

The optimal biomechanics during deep squatting require the pelvis to go into relative posterior rotation (relative to the neutral or anterior pelvic tilt position), and the lumbar spine to move into flexion (again relative to the neutral lordotic curve). If the individual has optimal psoas function, with a balance existing between their

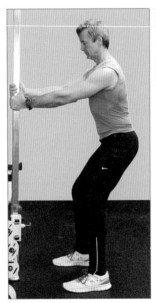 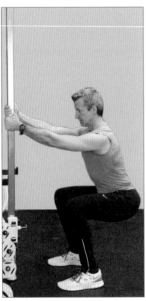 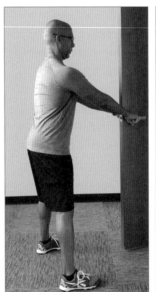 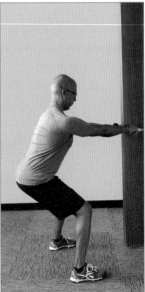

Supported Squat—machine (left images) and doorway (right images). The individual grasps lightly for support so that they are able to relax and sit back into their hips while maintaining TPC alignment during the pattern.

Clinical Consideration: A Note About Hip Restriction

A qualified health care practitioner can determine whether or not an individual's loss of hip range of motion is secondary to myofascial or capsular restrictions. Myofascial restrictions often occur secondarily to gripping (excessive contraction) around the hip complex. While any muscle can be over-contracted, clinically the most common muscles treated include the superficial gluteus maximus, posterior fibers of gluteus medius, deeper hip rotators, rectus femoris, and tensor fasciae latae.

While restriction may happen secondary to trauma or surgery, capsular restrictions can occur from years of chronic myofascial restrictions and/or gripping as noted above. Various release strategies—including manual therapy, self-myofascial release, cuing, and Mindful Release™—will often help restore resting myofascial tone and hence capsular mobility.

Once the restriction has been released, it is important to retrain the individual in a movement pattern that helps activate the psoas and related hip muscles while using the new range of motion, so that a new neuromotor pattern can be established. The Supported Squat is a great pattern for activating the psoas (and the rest of the DMS), while grooving the hips through their new range of motion.

---

superficial and deep myofascial systems, and they can control their joint positions, generally there are no problems with performing a deep squat. In fact, deep squatting then becomes an excellent way to stretch and mobilize the spine and hips.

To date there is insufficient evidence as to the psoas' role during the deep squat. On the basis of the working theory presented in this book, the likely function of the psoas during the deep squat is to:

- control the amount of spinal flexion during the lower ranges of the pattern;
- maintain hip centration throughout the pattern;
- work with the other muscles of the DMS to control segmental motion of the spine, the pelvis and sacroiliac joints, and the hips.

While in theory everyone should be able to perform deep squats, there are a multitude of

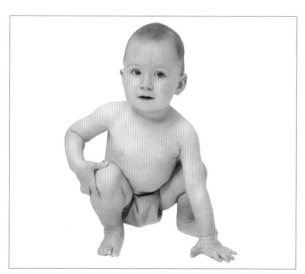

Deep squatting—optimal alignment and control with appropriate soft tissue mobility enables the baby to safely deep squat.

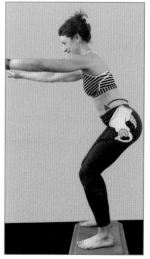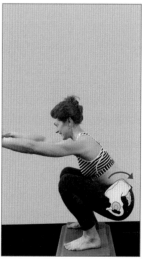

Deep squatting—during early to mid ranges, the pelvis should move anteriorly while the lumbar spine remains neutral (lordotic) (left image). During late to end ranges, the pelvis will gradually rotate posteriorly and the lumbar spine will flex (right image).

factors that prohibit many individuals in modern society from safely doing so. These reasons include (but are not limited to):

- Hip joint restrictions secondary to excessive myofascial tone or gripping in the posterior hip muscles and/or degenerative joint changes
- Joint degeneration in the pelvis, knees, and/or ankle and feet
- Loss of ankle and/or foot mobility
- Non-optimal breathing strategy and decreased ability to suspend and control the thorax over the pelvis
- Excessive myofascial tone or gripping in the hip, back, and/or abdominal regions
- Non-optimal control and excessive gripping (increased tone) of the pelvic floor
- Many years of sitting in chairs, often beginning in the developmental years
- Sedentary lifestyle

Many individuals who are encouraged to perform deep squatting do not have the requisite range of motion (ROM) or control required to safely load their joints in this position. Unless the individual possesses the requisite ROM and the ability to control their TPC and lower extremity, deep squatting will simply drive compensations during the pattern.

Common compensations include:

- Excessive posterior pelvic rotation and lumbar spine flexion
- Excessive flexion in the mid to lower thoracic spine
- Overstretching of the posterior sacroiliac joint ligaments
- Excessive knee abduction and foot pronation (or supination), and overstretching of the soft tissues of the medial knee and foot
- Excessive external hip rotation

For many individuals, especially the general population, repetitive deep squatting as an exercise—especially under external load—is contraindicated. Squatting to a position where the TPC and lower extremities remain neutrally aligned and controlled is a much safer and more effective method for gaining the benefits, without incurring the risks associated with a deeper squatting pattern. However, if an individual has optimal mechanics (alignment, breathing, and control of their TPC and hip complex) and can maintain these throughout the pattern, they can safely add the Deep Squat to their program.

Split Squat

The Split Squat pattern is a prerequisite for lunging, as the alignment and mechanics at the end of the lunge are essentially the same as those for the Split Squat. The individual must be able to maintain their alignment and control while performing the Split Squat before progressing to the Forward Lunge.

While the Split Squat is generally considered a progression for some individuals who struggle with the squatting pattern, it can actually be the preferred way to teach them how to align and control their TPC and use their hips, since they are focused on one side (the forward leg) at a time.

Setting Up the Split Squat Pattern

- The individual starts with their legs about hip-width apart to the side, and initially split front to back about 3–4 feet. Their front foot should be supported in a tripod fashion, meaning that most of the pressure will be under the first joint (or big-toe side of the foot), the fifth joint (or little-toe side of the foot), and the heel. The hip, knee, ankle, and foot should be aligned with each other so that a straight line goes from the hip joint, through the inside to middle of the knee joint, and to a point between the first and second digits of the foot. Their rear foot should be supported on the metatarsophalangeal joints, with the heel

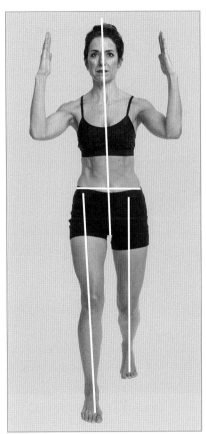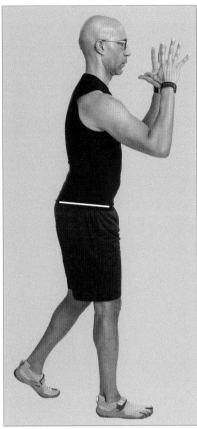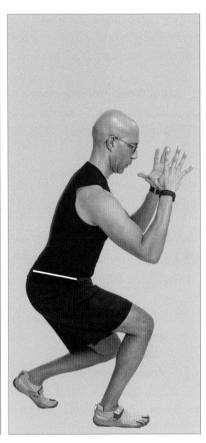

Split Squat—alignment of TPC and lower extremities (left); the pelvis should remain neutral at the beginning (middle) and ending positions (right) of the pattern.

slightly raised. The hip, knee, ankle, and foot of this leg should also be aligned. Since the aim is to focus primarily on the front leg, approximately 60–80% of their weight will be on that leg, with the remaining 20–40% on the rear leg.

- The individual aligns their trunk over their pelvis—essentially they are stacking their TPC. They should be in a relatively neutral spinal alignment, and the lower opening of the rib cage should face toward their feet and not forward. Throughout the pattern, the pelvis should remain in an anterior pelvic tilt, with their ASISs slightly anterior to, or in front of, their pubic symphysis.

- The first movement in the Split Squat pattern should be a hip hinge, or flexion of the hips, which moves the pelvis posteriorly. This movement will in turn create knee flexion and ankle dorsiflexion. As the individual lowers their body, they should be able to keep their

TPC stacked and their pelvis relatively neutral until all their available hip flexion is used up. To reduce overloading the spine, the majority of individuals only squat within the range through which they are able to maintain neutral pelvic and spine alignment. As in the Squat pattern above, the initial goal is to teach the individuals to control neutral alignment and master this position through a smaller range of motion, before they begin moving through a greater range.

- The individual returns to the top of the pattern in exactly the same TPC alignment.

As with the Squat pattern, the individual should be encouraged to sit back into their hips (eccentrically lengthening their glutes), lift their pelvis up toward the ceiling (concentrically shortening their glutes), and just allow their glutes to work, without encouragement to over-activate them at the end of the pattern. Excessive focus on glute contraction at the end of the Split Squat will tend to posteriorly rotate the pelvis and drive the femoral head anteriorly within the acetabulum.

If required, the individual can also use a machine, door handle, and/or suspension straps for support as demonstrated previously in the parallel squat pattern.

For demonstration of the Split Squat pattern, visit www.IIHFE.com/the-psoas-solution.

Common Signs of Dysfunction in the Split Squat

As with the Squat pattern, common signs of non-optimal control include:

- beginning or moving early into a posterior pelvic tilt and/or lumbar spine flexion;
- not maintaining TPC alignment or a level pelvis;
- losing alignment of the lower extremity.

The strategies and cues for improving the Split Squat pattern will be exactly the same as those given for the Squat pattern.

Another common issue during the Split Squat is frontal and/or transverse plane movement of the pelvis during the lowering phase of the pattern. As the individual lowers in the Split Squat, the pelvis can:

- laterally tilt in the frontal plane—the pelvis will tend to be higher on one side and lower on the other (image above right);
- rotate in the transverse plane—the innominate (one half of the pelvis) may anteriorly tilt (rotate) on one side and posteriorly tilt (rotate) on the other;
- both laterally tilt and rotate—there will be a combination of lateral tilt and rotation.

These pelvic deviations commonly occur with posterior myofascial tightness or capsular

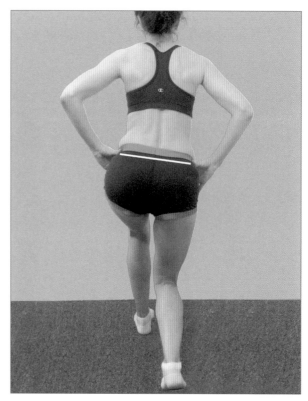

Lateral pelvic tilt is common during the Split Squat pattern when the individual is unable to sit back into their hip.

restriction of the hip. As noted earlier, myofascial release either manually or with an apparatus can help alleviate myofascial restrictions, while joint mobilization can help improve capsular restrictions. The individual is then cued as per previous recommendations, including "Release your posterior hip," "Let go around your hip," "Sit back into your hip," "Visualize the ball (femoral head) sinking back into the socket (acetabulum)," and "Let your sits bones go wide" to simultaneously improve hip flexion and leveling of the pelvis.

Supported Split Squat

Similarly to the Supported Squat, the Supported Split Squat can help groove the mechanics required for the traditional pattern. The individual can grasp a machine, the doorknobs of an open door, or suspension straps, and/or simply place their hands on the wall for support. All the mechanics and cues from above can be incorporated into the pattern.

Split Squat with Elevated Rear Leg

Once the individual has mastered the Split Squat pattern and can perform it, elevating the rear leg is the next progression. Because there is greater load when elevating the rear leg, for most individuals, this pattern is an excellent and generally safer alternative for loading the lower extremity as well as the trunk and spine than performing barbell loaded the back squat. All the mechanics from the Supported Split Squat will be incorporated into this pattern.

Setting Up the Split Squat with Elevated Rear Leg Pattern

- The individual starts with their feet together and aligns their trunk over their pelvis— essentially they are stacking their TPC. They should be in a relatively neutral spinal alignment, and the lower opening of the rib cage should face toward their feet and not forward. The pelvis should be in an anterior pelvic tilt, with the ASISs slightly anterior to the pubic symphysis.
- Next, on the side which they will be working first, the foot should be supported in tripod fashion—most of the pressure will be under the first joint (or big-toe side of the foot), the fifth joint (or little-toe side of the foot), and the heel. The hip, knee, ankle, and foot should be aligned with each other so that a straight line goes from the hip joint, through the inside to middle of the knee joint, and to a point between the first and second digits of the foot (see image right).

  The individual then elevates and supports their rear foot on a step or bench, or over a bar. The hip, knee, ankle, and foot of this leg should also be aligned with each other. Similar to the Split Squat, the aim is to focus primarily on working the individual's forward leg: initially,

approximately 60–80% of their weight will be on that leg, with the remaining 20–40% on the rear leg. Eventually, only minimal weight should be supported by the rear leg, the ultimate goal being to maintain 90–95% of the bodyweight over the forward leg.

- The first movement in the pattern will be exactly the same as in the Split Squat—a hip hinge, or flexion of the hips. This movement will in turn create knee flexion and ankle dorsiflexion. As the individual lowers their body, they should be able to keep their TPC stacked and their pelvis relatively neutral until all their available hip flexion is used up. Their lower extremity should remain aligned— hip, knee, ankle, and foot—throughout the pattern.

  As previously, they should lower themselves only to as far as they are able to maintain

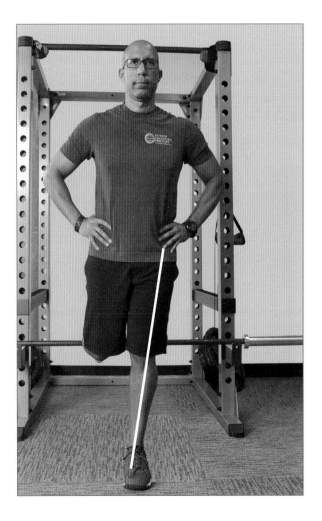

neutral pelvic alignment and therefore neutral spinal alignment. This is a great pattern for picking up deficiencies in the range of motion and control of hip flexion; the pelvis and/or lower extremity will deviate from neutral on the side with limited range and/or control.

- The individual returns to the top of the pattern in exactly the same TPC alignment. As with the Squat and Split Squat patterns, the individual should be encouraged to sit back into their hips (eccentrically lengthening their glutes), lift their pelvis up toward the ceiling (concentrically shortening their glutes), and just allow their glutes to work, without encouragement to over-activate them at the end of the pattern. As mentioned in the earlier patterns, excessive glute contraction at the end of the Split Squat with Elevated Rear Leg will tend to posteriorly rotate the pelvis and drive the femoral head anteriorly within the acetabulum.

As with the other squatting patterns, the Split Squat with Elevated Rear Leg can be progressed by loading with a medicine ball, dumbbells, or kettle bells.

For demonstration of the Elevated Rear Leg Split Squat pattern, visit www.IIHFE.com/the-psoas-solution.

Single Leg Squat

Setting Up the Single Leg Squat Pattern

The Single Leg Squat Pattern is the final Squat progression. It is an excellent way to load the lower extremity without the risk of overloading the spine which often occurs with barbell loaded variations of the squat pattern. It is a very sport-specific functional progression of the squatting pattern since nearly every sport requires single leg strength and stability.

Proper performance however requires tremendous strength and coordination to maintain the optimal mechanics throughout the pattern. The individual should be able to easily maintain alignment and control while in single leg stance for a minimum of 30 seconds and without significant gripping prior to performing the Single Leg Squat.

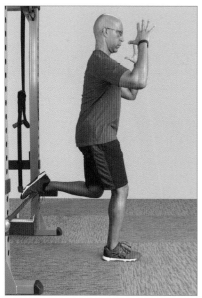 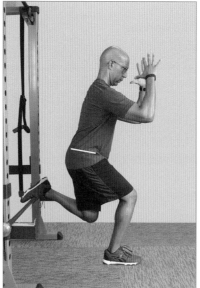 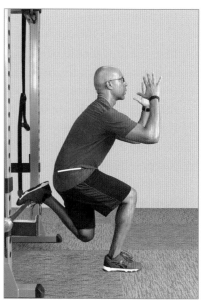

Elevated Rear Leg Split Squat—Neutral alignment (left and middle images); posterior pelvic tilt and lumbar spine flexion often occurs when the individual is no longer able to maintain adequate anterior pelvic tilt and is moving beyond their range of motion and/or level of control (image right).

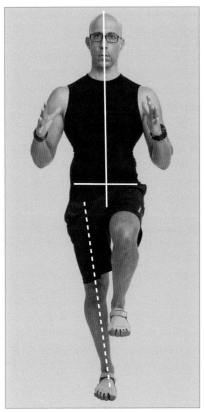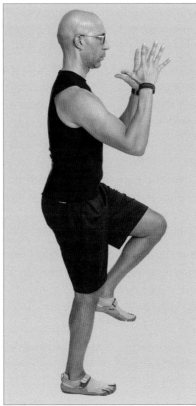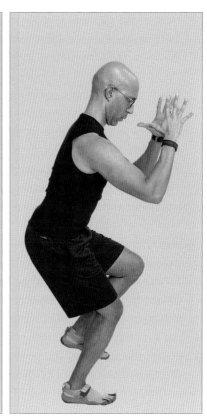

Single Leg Squat—optimal alignment in Single Leg Stance (above left); maintain TPC and lower extremity alignment during the Single Leg Squat (middle and right images).

All the mechanics discussed previously will apply to the Single Leg Squat:

- The TPC will remain aligned and stacked
- The hip, knee, and ankle-foot will remain aligned
- The foot tripod remains stable and controlled

As with the previous patterns, the individual begins with a slight hip hinge and sits back into their hip while maintaining TPC and lower extremity alignment. They will only lower themselves to the point where they are able to maintain neutral alignment and control. They should not over-grip the glutes at the top of the pattern.

Once the individual can flawlessly perform 20 or more repetitions, they can load the pattern with dumbbells, medicine balls, or kettlebells.

Deadlift

There are many variations of the Deadlift pattern one can perform. The traditional version of the deadlift pattern which will be discussed below works primarily the same movement pattern and muscles as the squat pattern. Besides the position of the load, the greatest difference between the deadlift and squat is the amount of forward lean of the TPC; the TPC tends to be more upright during a squat and angled further forward during a deadlift.

Setting Up the Deadlift Pattern

The individual may use a barbell, a trap or hex bar, kettlebells, or dumbbells to load the deadlift pattern.

- The individual starts with their feet about shoulder-width apart. The feet should be supported like a tripod, meaning that most of the pressure will be under the first metatarsophalangeal joint (or big-toe side of the foot), the fifth metatarsophalangeal joint (or little-toe side of the foot), and the calcaneus (heel). The hip, knee, ankle, and foot should be aligned with each other so that a straight line goes from the hip joint, through the inside to middle of the knee joint, and to a point between the first and second digits of the foot.

- The individual aligns their trunk over their pelvis—essentially they are stacking their TPC. They should be in a relatively neutral spinal alignment, and the lower opening of their rib cage should face toward their feet and not forward. The pelvis should be neutrally aligned (anterior pelvic tilt), with their ASISs slightly anterior to (in front of) their pubic symphysis. An ability to achieve this alignment is a good indication that the psoas is functioning properly. Their core (TPC) should be activated or 'braced' to maintain stability during the pattern.

- The individual lowers their body to grasp the bar—this movement should be similar to a hip hinge, or flexion of the hips, which rotates the pelvis into further anterior pelvic tilt.

To facilitate a safer deadlifting position for the spine and pelvis, the goal should be to use a range through which the individual is able to maintain neutral pelvic and spine alignment.

For individuals lacking the requisite range of motion required to lower their body to the floor without posteriorly rotating their pelvis or over-flexing their lumbar spine, place steps under the weights or use a rack to raise the level to which the individual can still maintain neutral alignment.

- The individual lifts out of the bottom of the pattern to stand upright and maintain neutral TPC alignment. They should be using (but not over-contracting) their glute complex (gluteus maximus, medius, and minimus) and hamstrings to rise from the bottom position. To avoid overloading the spine (facet joints), the erector spinae should be isometrically contracting and not actively extending during the pattern.

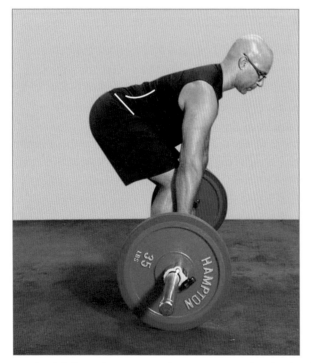 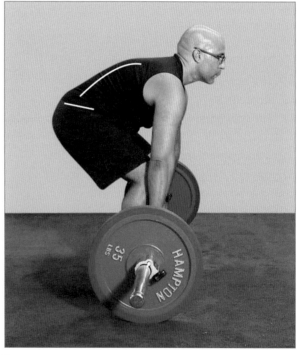

Optimal (left) and non-optimal set up pattern for the deadlift pattern. To reduce overloading the lumbar spine, the pelvis should be anteriorly tilted and the lumbar spine should be relatively neutral (left image) versus the pelvis being posteriorly tilted with excessive spinal flexion (right image).

As with the Squat pattern, a common cue is to instruct individuals to activate, or "squeeze," their glutes at the top of the pattern. However, as discussed earlier, this cue tends to cause the pelvis to posteriorly rotate, the lumbar spine to flex, and the femoral head to be driven excessively anteriorly within the acetabulum.

For demonstration of the Deadlift pattern, visit www.IIHFE.com/the-psoas-solution.

Please note: The suggestions noted throughout this section are referring to using the deadlift to train movements for everyday life and to reduce the stress upon the trunk, spine, and hip and thus do not necessarily apply to the sport of powerlifting. Due to the heavy loads that are utilized during heavy or maximal deadlifting, there may be a need to posteriorly translate the thorax in order to 'lock out' the lift.

To facilitate more optimal movement of the hip joint, while ensuring co-activation of the psoas and glutes, several of the cues discussed earlier are helpful during the Deadlift pattern as well:

- Individuals are encouraged to "sit back" with their hips (eccentrically lengthening the glutes and posterior hip complex) and cued to "spread," "lengthen," or "let go" during the lowering phase in order to ensure proper posterior glide of the femoral head within the acetabulum.
- Individuals are encouraged to lift their head up toward the ceiling (concentrically contracting the glutes and posterior hip complex), allowing their glutes to work, but without encouragement to over-activate and/or "squeeze" them at the end of the pattern. An effective cue is to "lift the head toward the ceiling" to ensure that they are maintaining neutral alignment, rather than translating their pelvis forward. This strategy also helps maintain optimal length and tension in the psoas and other spinal stabilizers.

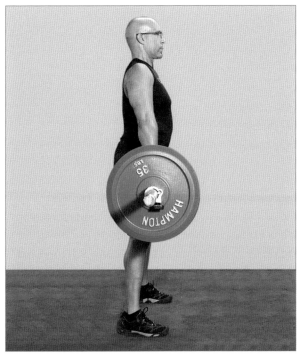 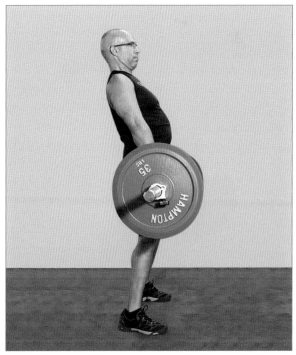

Optimal ending position of the deadlift pattern (left image)—the individual is cued to stand tall or drive the top the head towards the ceiling. Non-optimal ending position (right image)—the individual over-extends his back thereby overloading the spine and over-grips his glutes which drive his pelvis in posterior pelvic tilt.

Clinical Consideration: Knee Dominant Versus Hip Dominant Patterns

The strength and conditioning industry commonly refers to deadlift and squat patterns as *'knee-dominant'* movements meaning both the hip and knees are flexing so there is relatively equal contribution between the glutes, hamstrings and quadriceps. The Stiff-Legged variation of the Deadlift pattern, which will be discussed in the bending chapter, would be considered more of a *'hip-dominant'* pattern since the movement primarily occurs around the hip joint and is therefore targeting the glutes and posterior chain musculature.

Much of the general population (including athletes as well) have a poor ability to anteriorly rotate their pelvis to appropriately load the glutes and posterior hip complex; hence the preponderance of individuals being categorized as having 'weak' or 'amnesic' glutes. Therefore, regardless of whether a pattern is considered knee-dominant (Squats, Lunges, Step Ups, Traditional Deadlifts, etc.) or hip-dominant (Stiff-Legged Deadlifts, Bridges, Reaches, etc.) the emphasis is always on trying to maximize loading the glutes and posterior hip musculature while ensuring the psoas as part of the DMS stabilizes the trunk, spine, pelvis, and hip complex throughout the pattern. Therefore, whether the knees are bending during the pattern or not, all lower extremity patterns are considered hip-dominant movements.

Throughout the Deadlift pattern, be sure to monitor for compensations similar to those noted during the Squat pattern. The corrections will be similar for the deadlift pattern as were used during the squat pattern.

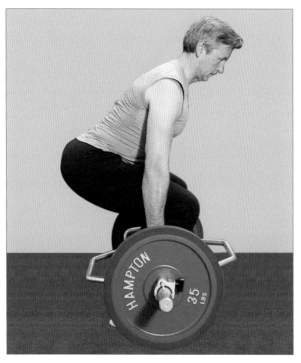

The Deadlift pattern performed with the Hex Bar: The benefit of using a hex bar is that it allows for a more natural loading position of the shoulders and brings the load closer to the individual's center of mass (core) and base of support (feet). The downside of using the hex bar is that many individuals will assume a narrower stance which can limit their ability to anteriorly rotate their pelvis and will over-adduct their knees so that the bar doesn't hit the outside of their legs. If the individual has optimal alignment and control using the hex bar this is generally the preferred method for loading this pattern.

Summary of Psoas Function in Squatting and Deadlifting Patterns

At the trunk, spine, and pelvis

- Stabilizes the TLJ, lumbar spine, and pelvis.
- Maintains neutral alignment of the TPC during most variations of the squatting and deadlifting patterns.
- Eccentrically controls spinal flexion and helps to maintain pelvic stability during the deep squat.

At the hip

- Centrates the femoral head within the acetabulum throughout the squatting and deadlifting patterns.
- Assists hip flexion by stabilizing the femoral head within the acetabulum during the eccentric or lowering phases of the patterns.
- Helps control excessive hip extension at the end of the concentric phase of the patterns.

Summary: Squatting and Deadlifting

1. During all variations of the squatting and deadlifting patterns, the psoas functions as a stabilizer of the spine and pelvis, so that the TPC remains in neutral alignment. In particular, the psoas stabilizes and anchors the TLJ, lumbar spine, and pelvis to help maintain integrity of the TPC.

2. The psoas axially compresses (stiffens) the lumbar spine, which helps maintain lumbar lordosis during the squatting and deadlifting patterns.

3. The psoas works with the lower fibers of the gluteus maximus to maintain femoral head centration within the acetabulum during the eccentric or lowering phase of the Squat and Deadlift patterns (as the hips are flexing). This enables the hips to remain centrated, which directly contributes to the ability to maintain the pelvis in a neutral (anterior pelvic tilt) and level position through the early to mid phases of the patterns (as well as during the progressions).

Signs of non-optimal psoas function during the squatting and deadlifting patterns:

- Loss of lumbar lordosis when beginning or initially lowering into the patterns.
- Lack of posterior glide of the femoral head, resulting in early and/or excessive spinal flexion and posterior pelvic rotation during the lowering phase of the patterns.
- Excessive extension at the TLJ early in the lowering phase of the patterns.
- Unleveling (frontal plane motion) and/or rotation (transverse plane motion) of the pelvis during any point of the pattern.
- Excessive anterior translation of the femoral head, posterior pelvic tilt, and/or lumbar spine flexion at the end of the concentric phase of the pattern.

Lunging

Introduction

The lunging pattern is one of the most versatile of the fundamental patterns for lifting things from the ground. It is not always necessary and/or practical to lift moderate to heavy objects from the ground using the squatting pattern. On these occasions, the lunge provides an alternative to the squat for lifting things from the ground and returning to the upright position. Additionally, when performed in multiple planes of motion, it is an excellent pattern for mobilizing the hips and lower extremities. The lunge is also a great pattern for developing lower body coordination for sport or recreational activities.

Additional benefits of the lunging pattern include:

- It trains alignment and control of the trunk, spine, and pelvis, in addition to the lower extremities in the upright position.
- It is an effective method for lengthening the psoas and hip flexors of the rear leg.
- A reaching version of the lunge is one of the most efficient methods for quickly picking up objects of moderate weight from the ground, and returning to the upright position.
- When performed in three dimensions, it is an excellent pre-activity or functional warm-up pattern for mobilizing the lower extremities.
- When loaded with weights—barbells, dumbbells, kettlebells, etc.—the lunge becomes an excellent exercise pattern for conditioning the core (the thoracopelvic cylinder—TPC).
- It can be used to train specific movements required for certain sports, including (but not limited to) tennis, basketball, and baseball.
- When performed in a rapid manner, or in combination with overhead presses, chops, and other exercise patterns, the lunge becomes an excellent tool for metabolic conditioning.

Psoas' Role in the Lunging Pattern

In many ways, psoas function in the lunging pattern is exactly the same as in the Split Squat pattern. There are three primary ways in which the psoas contributes to an optimal lunging pattern:

1. The psoas stabilizes the lumbar spine, which helps to maintain lumbar lordosis and thereby prevent excessive spinal flexion (flattening of the lumbar spine). Additionally, the psoas helps to maintain a neutral pelvis position (anterior pelvic tilt) during the lunging pattern.
2. In the lead leg, the psoas and lower glutes help centrate the femoral head within the acetabulum, ensuring optimal hip flexion (hip hinge) and maintenance of neutral pelvic and spinal alignment during the lunging pattern. Optimal hip centration helps to maintain the neutral position of the pelvis throughout the pattern.
3. The psoas eccentrically lengthens to prevent spinal extension, anterior innominate rotation, and hip extension in the rear, or trailing, leg.

Breathing Strategy During the Lunging Pattern

Similar to the squatting patterns, there are two general breathing strategies that will be used during the lunging patterns discussed in this chapter:

1. The individual inhales as they step out and lower into the lunge, and exhales as they push back to the starting position.
2. The individual inhales prior to the start of the repetition, exhales as they lower, and inhales as they push back to the starting position.

Choose the breathing strategy that enables your client to be most successful in maintaining optimal alignment and control during the pattern.

Forward Lunge

Essentially, the Forward Lunge is a dynamic version of the Split Squat pattern; therefore proficiency in the Split Squat pattern is required before performing any version of the lunging pattern. Since the mechanics are very similar between the two patterns, the individual must be able to maintain alignment and control while performing the Split Squat before they are progressed to the Forward or Reverse versions of the pattern.

The discussion that follows will focus on maintaining neutral alignment of the TPC (thorax stacked over the pelvis, lumbar lordosis, and anterior pelvic rotation) throughout the lunging pattern. The individual will therefore only be lunging to a length and depth that allows them to maintain neutral alignment of the TPC and lower extremity.

Setting Up the Forward Lunge Pattern

- The individual begins by standing with their legs about hip-width apart, their TPC in neutral alignment, and their weight on their feet tripods (see top left image, opposite page).
- They step forward with one leg and land on their foot tripod, while simultaneously decelerating the motion by flexing their hip, knee, and ankle and maintaining alignment and control—this is the loading position of the pattern. In this position the individual should be maintaining the same TPC alignment (the thorax stacked over the pelvis, and a neutral, level position of the pelvis) as in the start position.
  In the forward leg, their lower extremity should be aligned in such a way that a straight line passes from their hip, through the medial aspect of their knee, and to a point between digits one and two of their front foot (see top right image, opposite page). There should be no excessive sway or loss of body control in this position. Virtually all their bodyweight should be over the forward leg at this point.

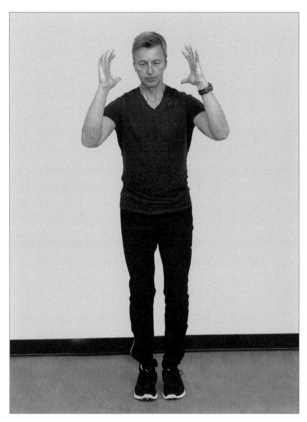 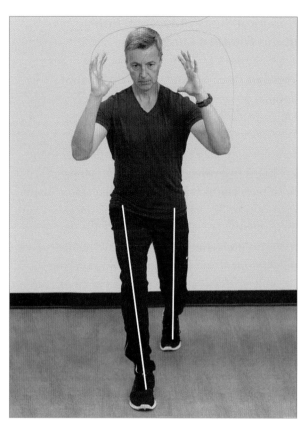

The Lunge pattern—beginning (left image); end (right image).

Their rear, or trailing, leg should be aligned as well—a straight line should pass through their hip, knee, and foot—and the ankle should be in plantar flexion, with the heel off the ground.

- To return to the starting position, there should be a combination of hip and knee extension, with the emphasis on using the hip rather than primarily extending the knee. Using the gluteal complex and hamstring of the forward leg, the individual pushes themselves back to the starting position, with no change in their alignment.

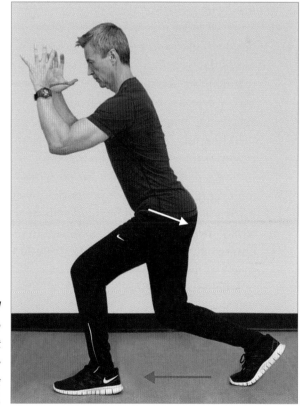

The Forward Lunge—The TPC remains aligned throughout the pattern and the individual only lowers to the point where they can maintain neutral alignment of the pelvis (anterior pelvic tilt) and lumbar spine lordosis (image right). The individual focuses on sitting into his front hip (arrow) as he lunges forward.

Common Signs of Dysfunction in the Forward Lunge

There are three common signs that indicate non-optimal psoas involvement during the Forward Lunge pattern:

1. *Non-optimal TPC alignment at the beginning.* Many individuals begin their lunging pattern in a posterior pelvic tilt and lumbar spine flexion position. To ensure activation of the psoas and deep myofascial system (DMS), the individual must understand how to achieve neutral pelvic alignment and how to maintain it during the lunging pattern. Have the individual palpate their anterior superior iliac spine (ASIS) and pubic symphysis: the ASIS should be slightly anterior to their pubic symphysis.
   Rib cage suspension—essentially lifting the thorax up and over the pelvis—is also an effective strategy for achieving neutral pelvic alignment. Review rib cage suspension in Appendix III.

2. *Non-optimal TPC alignment at various points in the lunging pattern.*
   a. *Posterior pelvic tilt and/or lumbar spine flexion in the loading position.* During an ideal lunging pattern, the pelvis should remain in neutral (anterior tilt). This range will be determined by the individual's specific hip range of motion and will therefore vary from person to person. Early posterior tilt and lumbar spine flexion indicates that the individual has posterior joint capsule restriction or posterior myofascial tension, and/or is not actively letting their hip muscles relax enough to ensure optimal hip centration. Restriction in any of these regions can compromise optimal psoas function.
   Self-myofascial release, manual therapy release, and/or verbal or tactile cuing can be effective in helping the individual release the areas they are holding and to maintain centration of the hips. Verbal cues, including "Sit your hips back," "Release from your posterior hips," "Let your sits bones go wide," and "Think of letting the ball sink back in the socket," can encourage more-ideal posterior femoral head glide. Activation of the psoas and other muscles of the DMS can additionally be effective in rebalancing the muscles around the hip and in reducing high levels of tone or gripping.
   For those who are new to the Forward Lunge pattern, and/or are relatively unsteady as they step out, the range of motion can be shortened so that they are either not stepping as far or sitting as deeply into the pattern. If they are struggling too much with their alignment and/or control, then have them return to the Split Squat pattern.
   b. *Lateral tilt of the pelvis.* As discussed in the section on the Split Squat, lateral tilting of the pelvis occurs when the individual does not have enough anterior pelvic rotation (hip flexion) and ends up tilting their pelvis laterally rather than maintaining pure sagittal plane motion (image below).

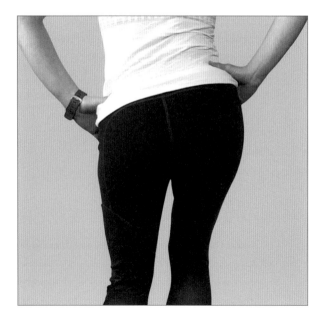

c. As with Split Squats, release the posterior hip and cue the individual in how to self-monitor and detect when they are losing neutral pelvic alignment. For most individuals, they will need to limit the range (depth) of the movement until they've gained better range of motion and control.

d. *Excessive extension at the thoracolumbar junction (TLJ) as they push back to the starting position.* Many individuals will step too far out and/or will not utilize the posterior hip complex (glutes and hamstrings) appropriately. As a consequence, they will hyperextend at their TLJ in order to return to the starting position (image right). In essence, rather than using their glutes to push themselves back, they are overusing their erector spinae muscles to shift their trunk, which will overstretch the psoas and abdominal wall and thereby perpetuate the dysfunction.

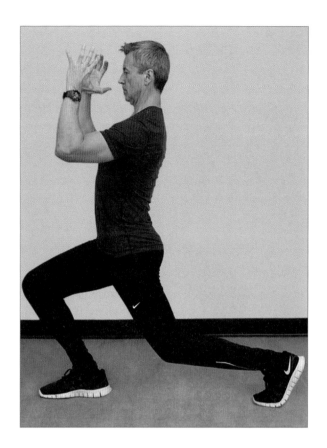

To improve TPC alignment, cue the client to lower their thorax so that it is stacked on top of their pelvis. A simple way to kinesthetically cue them into a more ideal TPC alignment is to have them place one hand over their lower abdomen and the other over their sternum, and maintain the distance between their hands throughout the pattern (image right).

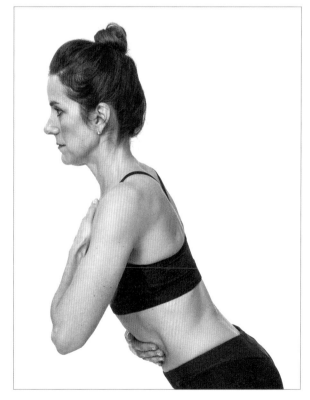

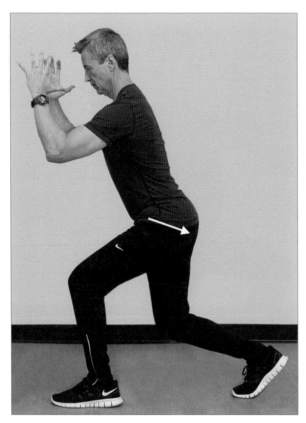 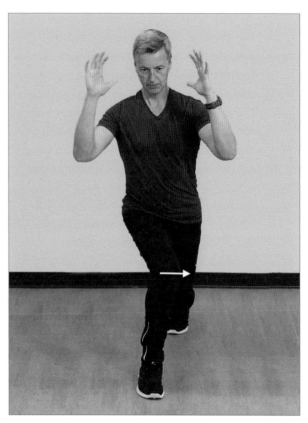

The Lunge pattern—optimal alignment (left image); increased valgus motion at the knee (right image).

Cuing them to sit or 'sink' into their front hip (arrow in image above) and then use their posterior hip muscles to push themselves back to the starting position is also helpful. Shortening the range and depth of motion can also help them develop the ability to use their forward leg, rather than relying upon trunk extension to return to the starting position.

3. *Non-optimal alignment of the lower extremity in the loading position.* While not always directly linked to a psoas issue, there are two common issues regarding the lower extremity that can in turn influence function of the psoas—either the individual's knee moves into excessive valgus position (image above right), or the knee moves too far forward over the front foot. Each of these issues can be related to the individual's experience with the pattern and/or with their TPC control. Proper instruction and appropriate cuing of the pattern usually corrects both of these issues:

a. Ensuring that the individual controls their TPC will often improve overall body control and hence alignment of the lower extremity. Use any of the previously mentioned cues.

b. Cuing the individual to sit back into their front hip helps keep them from shifting their bodyweight forward, and thus the knee from moving too far forward.

c. Optimal loading of the foot tripod—allowing the foot to spread while maintaining arch control—while sinking into the front hip will also encourage better lower extremity alignment.

Reverse Lunge

As the name implies, the movement in the Reverse Lunge pattern is essentially the reverse of that in the Forward Lunge pattern. Rather than stepping forward, the individual steps back while maintaining all the mechanics of the Forward Lunge pattern. Many clients actually find it easier to master flexion of the forward hip, while maintaining neutral pelvic alignment, when they use the Reverse Lunge rather than the Forward Lunge.

Setting Up the Reverse Lunge Pattern

- The individual begins by standing with their legs about hip-width apart, their TPC in neutral alignment, and their weight on their feet tripods.
- They step back with one leg while flexing the hip, knee, and ankle of the forward, or stationary, leg. As they lower their body, they should be maintaining the same TPC alignment as in the start position (the thorax stacked over the pelvis, and a neutral, level position of the pelvis).

In the loaded or end position, the lower extremity of their forward side should be aligned in such a way that a straight line passes from their hip, through the medial aspect of their knee, and to a point between digits one and two of their front foot. There should be no excessive sway or loss of body control in this position. Virtually all their bodyweight should be over the forward leg at this point, with less than 10% of their weight transitioning onto the rear leg.

Their rear, or trailing, leg should be aligned as well—a straight line should pass through their hip, knee, and foot—and the ankle should be in plantar flexion, with the heel off the ground.

- Using the gluteal complex, hamstrings, and quadriceps of the forward leg, they lift themselves up and over the stationary foot and return to the starting position. There should

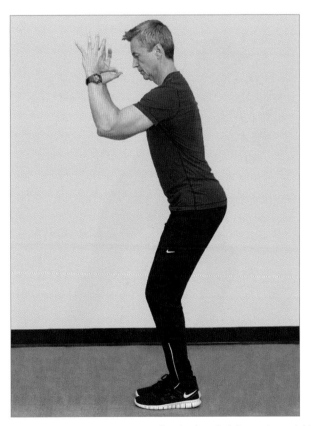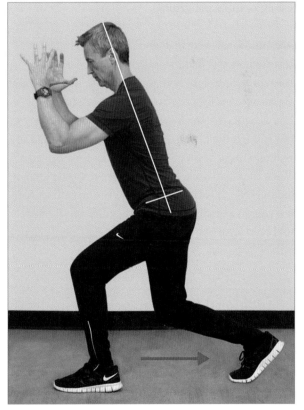

The Reverse Lunge pattern—beginning (left image); end (right image).

be no change in their TPC or lower extremity alignment throughout the pattern.

Similar to the Forward Lunge, increase the challenge by having the individual hold a medicine ball, dumbbells, a barbell, or kettlebells. Ensure that the load does not compromise the individual's alignment, breathing, and control during the pattern. The Reverse Lunge can also be progressed by taking a longer step, sinking deeper into the forward hip, and/or performing the repetitions at a faster pace.

Common Signs of Dysfunction in the Reverse Lunge

As with the previous patterns, common signs of non-optimal psoas control include loss of TPC alignment, loss of neutral alignment of the pelvis, non-optimal centration of the forward hip, and (indirectly) loss of lower extremity alignment. Use any of the previous strategies and cues covered in the Forward Lunge pattern to correct the individual's alignment and restore optimal patterning.

One additional issue that tends to arise with the Reverse Lunge is that the individual transfers too much of their weight onto their rear leg. This generally occurs because they are not maintaining enough of their weight over the forward leg, and not sinking into enough hip flexion on that side. Instruct them to maintain more of their weight over the forward leg. When they step back, have them take a shorter step, and only touch their rear toes onto the ground instead of trying to actually step back. They can also lightly hold onto a surface in order to maintain better balance as they focus on flexing their forward leg.

Additional Lunge Progressions

Once the individual has mastered the basic lunge, they can increase the challenge by using additional planes of motion (frontal and transverse plane lunge, right images) and/or load. Ensure that the plane of motion or load does not compromise the individual's alignment, breathing, and control during the pattern.

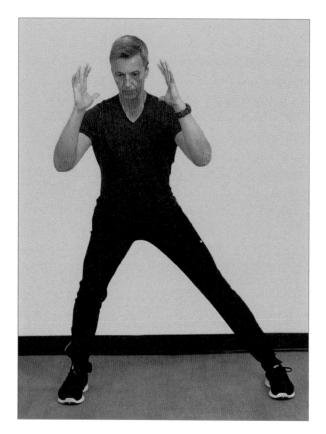

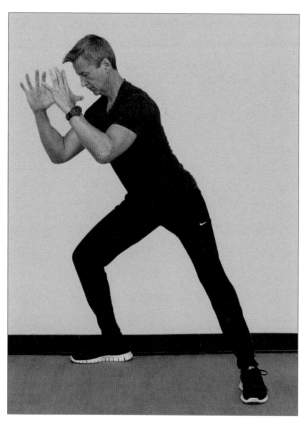

Frontal (top image) and transverse plane lunge (above) progressions.

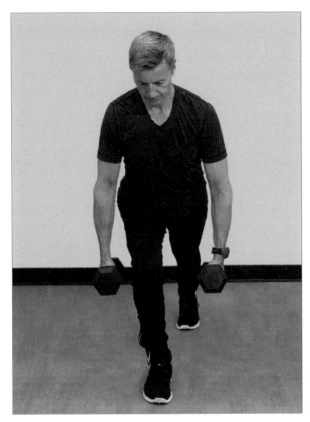 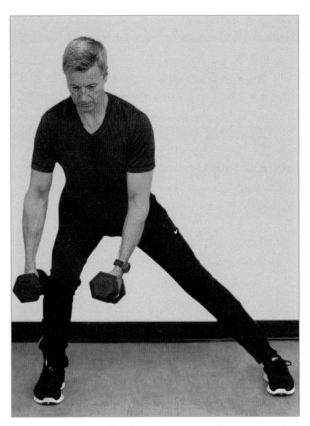

For additional challenge, add a reaching pattern and/or load. Ensure TPC as well as lower extremity alignment and control during the pattern.

Summary of Psoas Function in Lunging Patterns

At the trunk, spine, and pelvis
- Stabilizes the TLJ, lumbar spine, and pelvis.
- Maintains neutral alignment of the TPC during both the Forward Lunge and Reverse Lunge patterns.

At the hip
- Centrates the femoral head within the acetabulum throughout the lunging pattern.
- Assists hip flexion by stabilizing the femoral head within the acetabulum during the lowering or eccentric phase of the pattern.
- Helps control excessive hip and spine extension, as well as anterior rotation of the innominate in the rear leg.

Summary: Lunging

1. During the lunging pattern, the psoas functions as a stabilizer of the spine and pelvis, so that the TPC remains in neutral alignment. In particular, the psoas stabilizes and anchors the TLJ, lumbar spine, and pelvis to help maintain integrity of the TPC.

2. The psoas axially compresses (stiffens) the lumbar spine, which helps maintain lumbar lordosis during the lunging pattern.

3. The psoas works with the lower fibers of the gluteus maximus to maintain femoral head centration within the acetabulum during the lowering phase of the lunging pattern (as the hips are flexing). This enables the hips to remain centrated, which directly contributes to the ability to maintain the pelvis in neutral or anterior pelvic tilt.

Signs of non-optimal psoas function during the lunging pattern:

- Loss of lumbar lordosis when beginning or initially lowering into the pattern.
- Lack of posterior glide of the femoral head, resulting in spinal flexion and posterior pelvic rotation (and/or lateral tilt) during the lowering phase.
- Extension at the TLJ while returning from the Forward Lunge pattern.
- Unleveling (pelvic tilt in the frontal plane motion) and/or rotation (transverse plane motion) of the pelvis during any point of the pattern.
- Indirectly, contributes to the loss of lower extremity alignment in the forward leg during the loading phase.

Bending

Introduction

The ability to bend the trunk and spine is a functional requirement for nearly every activity in daily life. Bending forward to pick something up from the floor, lifting something overhead, or walking, for example, involve a certain degree of bending and contribution from the trunk, spine, pelvis, and/or hips.

When bending over to lift something that is fairly light from the floor or bottom shelf of a cabinet, it is not always necessary (and/or practical) to squat or lunge. In these cases, bending and/or hip hinging—another form of forward bending—can be safe and effective alternatives. Moving the arms overhead to reach a high shelf in the cabinet, throwing a ball, or lifting a child overhead all require the ability to extend or bend the spine backward. For efficient walking and running, the

spine and pelvis need to be able to bend forward and backward, as well as to the side, at different points of the gait cycle. It is easy to see the signs in an individual of an inability to optimally bend the spine, pelvis, and/or hips when they walk or run, as their gait appears very stiff and uncoordinated.

This chapter will look at various types of bending movement. The term "bending" incorporates several different movements (and sometimes a combination of movements) of the spine and/or pelvis-hip complex. The spine and pelvis-hip complex can bend in the following directions:

- *Forward*—in forward bending, where there is segmental movement of the vertebrae, the spine flexes and the pelvis anteriorly rotates over the femoral heads. When the thoracopelvic cylinder (TPC) is held stable, forward bending can also occur just at the hip joints by anteriorly rotating the pelvis over the femoral heads.
- *Side-to-side*—in side bending from the upright position, the spine laterally flexes and the pelvis remains relatively neutral or can laterally tilt (frontal plane motion).
- *Backward*—in backward bending, the spine extends and the pelvis posteriorly rotates

over the femoral heads. (The mechanics and use of the psoas in backward bending will be examined in Chapter 7.)

The reader is also referred to the discussion of relative hip movement in Chapter 1.

Psoas' Role in Bending Patterns

There are two primary ways in which the psoas contributes to bending:

1. *During forward bending*—the spine can flex or it can remain neutral:
    *   *With spinal flexion.* In this case the psoas will stabilize and contribute to segmental flexion of the lumbar spine. It helps ensure that each vertebral segment is contributing to the overall movement as the spine is flexing forward. While care should be taken to avoid the *end range*—the point in the range of motion where the muscles can no longer stabilize the joint—and repetitive movement, spinal flexion is a necessary pattern for stretching and mobilizing the posterior structures of the spine in individuals with a healthy spine.
    *   *With neutral spinal alignment.* Forward bending can be achieved by maintaining the TPC in neutral alignment and flexing only at the hip joints. Referred to as *hip hinging* or simply *hinging*, the pelvis anteriorly rotates over the stationary femoral heads. Essentially, hip hinging is closed-chain hip flexion, and the psoas will help stabilize the spine and pelvis, and then centrate the femoral heads within the acetabulum, so that flexion or hinging occurs strictly at the hip joint and not through flexion of the spine. If an individual suffers from low back pain, hip hinging is a safe pattern for them to use their hips and "spare the spine" (limit motion of the spine) when bending forward.

2. *During side bending*—from an upright position, the psoas may contribute to segmental lateral flexion of the spine; however, the muscle is more involved in decelerating the spine to avoid excessive joint compression on the side of bending. For example, in side bending to the right, the left psoas is eccentrically lengthening, while the right psoas is relatively passively shortening. However, if there is resistance to the motion, as when performing

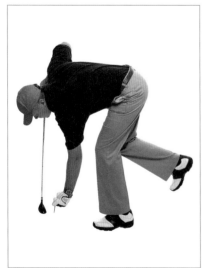 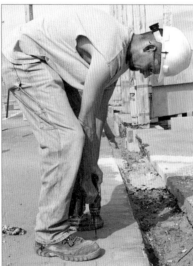 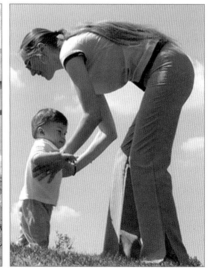

Various methods of forward bending—The golfer (left image) primarily uses a hip hinge bending pattern while the construction worker (middle image) utilizes primarily spinal flexion with very little contribution from his hips. The mother bending down to pick up her child (right image) uses a combination of hip hinge and spinal flexion.

Clinical Consideration: A Note About Spinal Flexion During Forward Bending

The amount of contribution from the hips in forward bending is dependent upon the load being lifted (the greater the load the less spinal flexion that should be used) and the individual's habits or how they've taught themselves to bend. Ideally during forward bending there should be a significant amount of anterior pelvic tilt to decrease the need for excessive amounts of spinal flexion.

While the spine should flex during forward bending there are some individuals who don't tolerate spinal flexion well and experience discomfort when in prolong spinal flexion; for example when sitting in a slumped posture or soft chair or when bending over to brush their teeth for example.

For those who are *flexion intolerant*—individuals who do not tolerate and experience dysfunction/

pain from bending forward with end range spinal flexion or maintaining their spine in a prolonged flexed position—keeping the spine in more neutral alignment is a safer method for repetitive forward bending tasks.

Clinically, it has been observed that a significant portion of the population has significant limitations in creating optimal anterior pelvic rotation (tilt) when they bend forward. Therefore, a significant part of most individual's training program is dedicated to improving their ability to anteriorly tilt their pelvis and while limiting the amount of spinal flexion. Generally spinal flexion is not trained until the individual demonstrates an optimal hip hinging strategy.

---

a unilateral carrying activity, the contralateral psoas is more likely to be actively assisting in maintaining a vertical position of the spine.

Training to Improve Bending

The following sections will describe the patterns designed to improve the use of the spine and pelvis-hip complex when bending:

- *Forward bending*—Forward Bend, Hip Hinge, and Roll-up patterns
- *Lateral, or side, bending*—Side Bend and Carrying patterns

Forward Bend

Since many activities of daily life and require forward bending, in individuals that aren't currently experiencing or have a history of spine issues associated with flexion it is useful to train them how to perform an optimal forward bend pattern. Generally when working with the general

population this pattern is performed only with body weight as the spinal risks associated with performing spinal flexion under excessive loads outweigh the benefits.

Setting Up the Forward Bend Pattern

- The individual starts with their feet about hip-width apart and their knees straight. Their weight should be supported on the feet tripods—most of the pressure will be under the first joint (or big-toe side of the foot), the fifth joint (or little-toe side of the foot), and the heel. The hip, knee, ankle, and foot should be aligned with each other, so that a straight line goes from the hip joint, through the middle of the knee joint, and to a point between the first and second digits of the foot.
- The individual aligns their trunk over their pelvis—essentially they are stacking their TPC. They should be in a relatively neutral spinal alignment, and the lower opening of the rib cage should face toward their feet and not forward. The pelvis should be in an

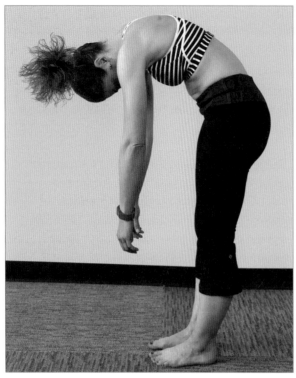 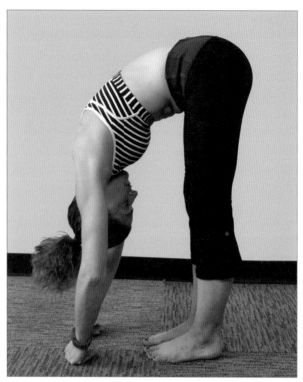

Forward Bending pattern—the individual begins with spinal flexion (left) and then continues bending forward by anteriorly tilting her pelvis (right). Ideally, most flexion during the forward bend pattern should occur at the hips rather than the spine.

anterior pelvic tilt, with their anterior superior iliac spines (ASISs) slightly anterior to their pubic symphysis.

- The individual begins gently flexing their head and neck by tucking their chin toward their chest and allowing slow, segmental flexion of their spine (image above left). It is important that the initial movement is slow, so that they can feel and control the movement of their spine as it flexes through the various regions.
- Once the individual has moved through lumbar spine flexion, they anteriorly rotate the pelvis in order to continue the forward bend movement (image above right).
- When they have achieved as much motion as they can without forcing their body into an end range of motion, the individual reverses the movement by first posteriorly rotating their pelvis, and then segmentally extending the lumbar, thoracic, and cervical spines. This is continued until they return to the starting position, with the TPC in neutral alignment.

Common Signs of Dysfunction in the Forward Bend

There are two common signs that indicate non-optimal psoas involvement during the Forward Bend pattern:

1. *Lack of segmental motion.* It is common for the thoracolumbar junction (TLJ) and/or the lumbar spine to remain in an extended position because the erector spinae muscles are hypertonic and maintaining the lordotic curve, and/or the psoas is inhibited and unable to contribute to flexing the spine.
2. *Inability to anteriorly rotate the pelvis.* This limitation arises when the superficial gluteus maximus, hamstrings, and/or superficial abdominal muscles are hypertonic. The individual will compensate by excessively flexing in either the thoracic or the lumbar spine. This postural and movement strategy will inhibit the psoas, overload the spinal discs and joints, and perpetuate faulty bending patterns.

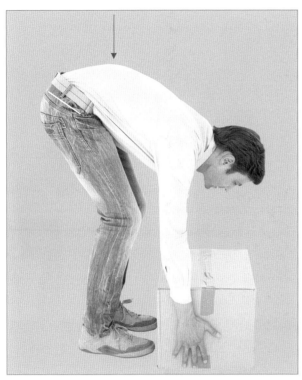

Non-optimal forward bend—the individual has decreased ability to anteriorly tilt his pelvis and therefore overflexes at his thoracolumbar region to compensate to reach the box.

Corrective Exercise Strategies for Improving the Forward Bend Pattern

- *Release and/or lengthen myofascial restrictions.* Self-myofascial release, manual therapy release, and similar strategies can be effective in releasing restrictions in the erector spinae (which limit segmental spinal flexion) or in the gluteus maximus, hamstrings, posterior hip musculature or abdominals (which limit anterior pelvic rotation). Follow up any releases with a pattern to improve psoas activation and segmental spinal and pelvic control— for example, the Pelvic Tilt (Chapter 2), Supported Squat (Chapter 4), or Hip Hinge Bridge (Chapter 7).

- *Self-monitor and limit pelvic motion.* Helping the individual self-monitor their own range of motion is the easiest method for training optimal pelvic movement:
  - The individual places their hands over their pelvis so that their thumbs are pointing toward their posterior superior iliac spines (PSISs), and their fingers are pointing toward their ASISs.
  - Their hands will be monitoring the movement of their pelvis as they flex their spine and then anteriorly rotate their pelvis. When they no longer feel the pelvis moving, they stop and reverse the pattern until they arrive back at the starting position. See Hip Hinge pattern overleaf.

- *Cue release and/or lengthening of myofascial restrictions.* The individual can be helped to release through the following regions:
  - Erector spinae—cue them to "let go" or "lengthen."
  - Back of their hips—cue them to "let go" or "lengthen," or to "send the tailbone long or behind them," to release through their glutes and/or hamstrings.

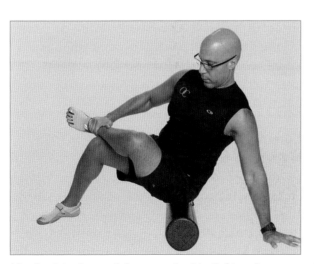
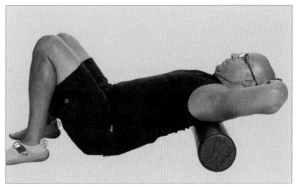

Myofascial release of the posterior hip (left) and erector spinae (right).

- Hip rotators—cue them to release or "widen" across their ischial tuberosities or sits bones.
- Abdominals—cue them to breathe into their belly to relax the abdominals as they anteriorly rotate their pelvis.

Hip Hinge

The Hip Hinge pattern is one of the fundamental patterns every client is taught because as noted above, so many individuals don't use their hips enough during forward bending. The inability to achieve enough anterior pelvic rotation (essentially this is the inability to flex the hips in the upright position) is one of the greatest contributors to overloading the lumbar spine. Because the spine remains neutral, the Hip Hinge pattern is one of the safest method for lifting heavier loads from a lower point.

Setting Up the Hip Hinge Pattern

- The individual begins in exactly the same alignment of their TPC and lower extremities as in the Forward Bend pattern. They place their hands upon their pelvis so they can monitor their own pelvic motion.
- The pattern is initiated by rotating pelvis anteriorly over the femoral heads. They anteriorly rotate their pelvis (tilt pelvis forward) as much as they can without losing alignment of their TPC or lower extremities (images above right). They should be cued to think 'long' (black arrow) from through the top of their head throughout the pattern.
- When there is no more available motion of the hips, the individual gently contracts their glutes and hamstrings in order to pull themselves back up to the starting position.
- While it is a common cue to instruct individuals to squeeze their glutes at the top of the Hip Hinge pattern, this will tend to posteriorly rotate the pelvis and drive the

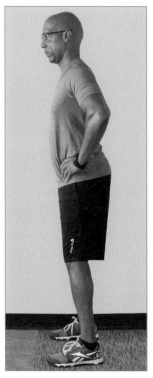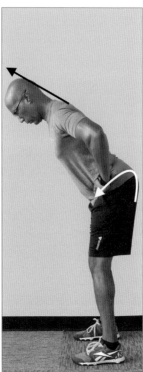

femoral head anteriorly within the acetabulum. The individual should maintain an active contraction; however, over-contraction of the glutes should be avoided as they return to the starting position.

For demonstration of the Hip Hinge pattern, visit www.IIHFE.com/the-psoas-solution.

Once the individual has mastered the Hip Hinge movement, they can be further challenged by loading them with a barbell (left and middle images opposite), dumbbells, or kettlebells. While the pelvis will translate or shift posteriorly, as with the body weight version, the pelvis should still anteriorly rotate (tilt forward) as the weight is lowered.

Common Signs of Dysfunction in the Hip Hinge

Frequently, individuals lack the stability in their lumbar spine and pelvis-hip complex, and/or lack appropriate length in their glutes, hamstrings, and posterior hip complex, to achieve a fully anteriorly

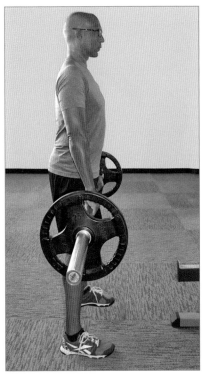 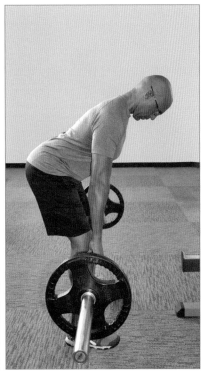 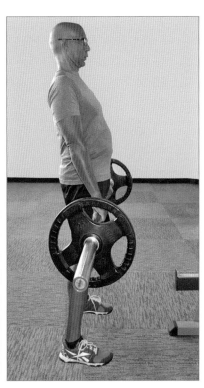

Hip Hinge pattern—beginning (left); end (middle); Over-extension of the thorax and posterior pelvic tilt (right) results when clients are cued to 'squeeze their glutes' or 'drive the pelvis forward' at the top of the pattern.

rotated pelvis. One of the most common signs that indicate non-optimal psoas involvement during the Hip Hinge pattern is the inability to achieve full anterior rotation of the pelvis and the individual will excessively flex at the lower lumbar spine.

Corrective Exercise Strategies for Improving the Hip Hinge Pattern

- *Improve the function of the psoas in the stabilization of the TPC and hip.* The Happy Baby and Modified Dead Bug progressions described in Chapter 4 can be helpful in restoring function of the psoas and in improving its function in the Hip Hinge pattern.
- *Self-monitor and limit pelvic motion.* Helping the individual self-monitor for movement of their pelvis is the easiest way to train optimal pelvic movement. See above for a description of how to teach self-monitoring of pelvic motion.

They can also perform a supported Hip Hinge, in which they place their hands on the wall and then focus on sitting back into their hips. The focus remains on rotating the pelvis forward (anterior) or over the femoral heads. Supported Hip Hinge: Optimal alignment in the Supported Hip Hinge pattern (left and middle images overleaf)—the individual is able to anteriorly rotate his pelvis and maintain a neutral spine alignment; Many individuals demonstrate poor ability to anteriorly tilt their pelvis and will compensate by over-flexing the spine (image right overleaf). Poor hip mobility or the decreased ability to move the pelvis anteriorly over the femoral heads is a common cause of low back pain and degenerative changes of the spine.

- *Release and/or lengthen myofascial restrictions.* Self-myofascial release, manual therapy release, and similar release strategies can be effective in releasing myofascial restrictions (in the superficial glutes, hamstrings, posterior hip rotators, abdominals) that are inhibiting the

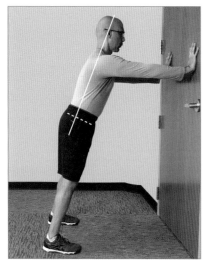
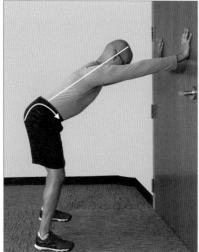
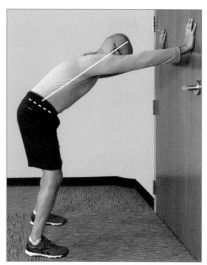

Supported Hip Hinge—beginning (left); end (middle); non-optimal anterior pelvic rotation and resultant lumbar spine flexion (right).

individual's ability to anteriorly rotate their pelvis. Follow up any release with a pattern to improve psoas activation and stabilization of the TPC—for example, the Happy Baby and/or Modified Dead Bug.

- *Cue release and/or lengthening of myofascial restrictions.* The individual can be cued to release through the back of their hips ("Lengthen through your glutes and hamstrings" and/or "Spread your ischial tuberosities apart") and/or through their abdominals (cue them to breathe into their belly while releasing any gripping) as they anteriorly rotate their pelvis.

Progressions

The Split Stance Hip Hinge is an excellent yet seldom used progression of the bilateral pattern. This pattern is an easy way to demonstrate asymmetries in forward bending between the individual's two sides. Similar to the bilateral version, initially the individual places their hands upon their pelvis to monitor pelvic rotation and only moves as far as they feel the pelvis rotating

(images below). As with the bilateral pattern this patterns can be loaded with dumbbells, kettlebells, barbells or cable machine.

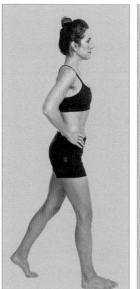
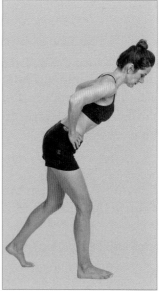

Split Stance Hip Hinge—the individual keeps her hands upon her pelvis so she is monitoring her pelvic rotation (tilt).

Once the individual demonstrates proficiency in the split stance version, they can be progressed to the single leg version of the Hip Hinge pattern. The individual should have an optimal Split

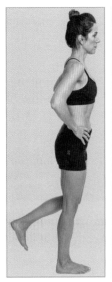
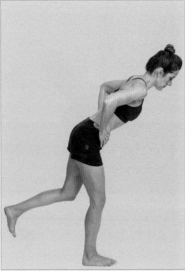

Single Leg Hip Hinge.

The individual must be able to maintain optimal alignment and control while in single leg stance prior to performing the hinging motion. Additionally, ensure that they maintain neutral alignment while anteriorly rotating their pelvis as they hinge forward (images top left).

For demonstration of the Split Stance and Single Leg variations of the Hip Hinge pattern, visit www.IIHFE.com/the-psoas-solution.

Single Leg Hip Hinge with Reach is a progression of the previous hinge patterns. Note the individual is able to maintain alignment as he reaches forward (left and middle images below). In individuals with poor hip dissociation, it is extremely common for them to rotate and/or laterally tilt their pelvis as they exceed the range of motion they are able to control (right image below). Performing the pattern in this manner will lead to the perpetuation of non-optimal movement patterns and is a common contributor to low back, pelvic, hip and knee issues.

Stance Hip Hinge and be able to maintain single leg stance without compensation for a minimum of 30 seconds per leg before progressing onto the single leg version. Ensuring optimal alignment and control in the single leg version is the prerequisite pattern to adding loading or reaching variations.

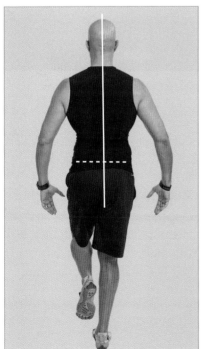
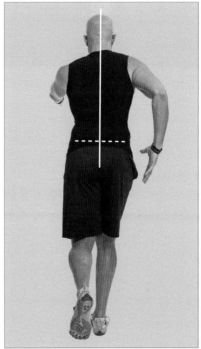
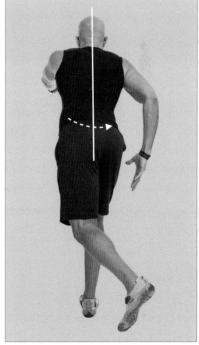

Single Leg Hip Hinge with Reach—TPC remains aligned as the individual hinges and reaches forward (left and middle images); many individuals will lose TPC alignment due to a poor Hip Hinge pattern and will compensate by rotating through their spine (right).

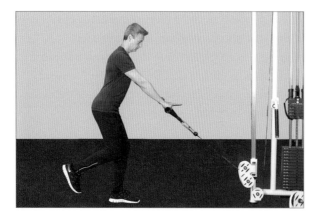
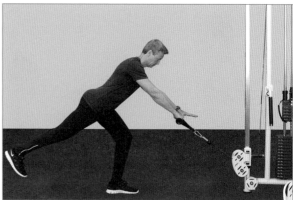
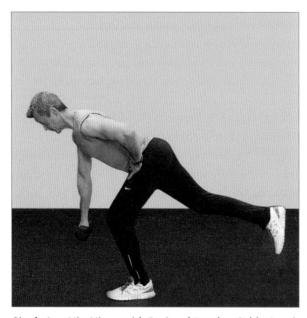
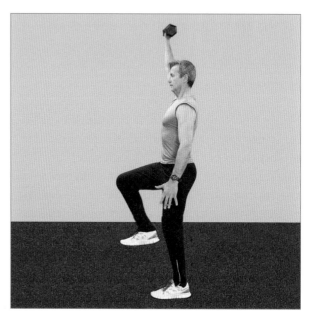

Single Leg Hip Hinge with Resisted Reach—Cable (top images) and dumbbell loaded (bottom images).

Single Leg Hip Hinge with Resisted Reach—the individual must be able to perform the Single Leg Hip Hinge with optimal alignment and control before moving on to loaded versions of the pattern. This pattern can be loaded with cables, dumbbells, or medicine balls. The mechanics are the same regardless of the loading pattern.

Roll-up

For individuals without a history of spinal pain or dysfunction, the Roll-up pattern is an effective exercise for training segmental spinal flexion and strengthening the abdominal wall in its role of spinal flexion. It helps coordinate the psoas and abdominal muscles in flexing the spine and can

be used as a fairly safe method for lengthening the muscles and fascia of the posterior chain.

Setting Up the Roll-up Pattern

- The individual lies on their back with their legs straight, and with their shoulders flexed so that the palms of their hands are facing the floor.

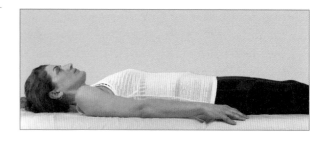

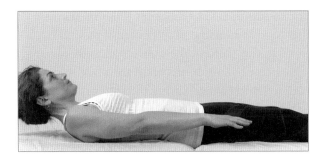 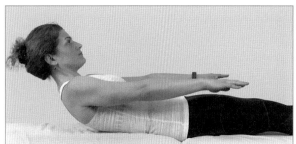

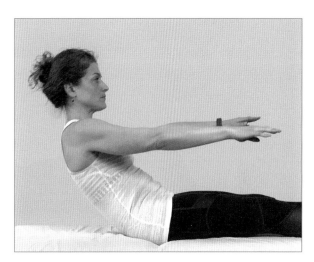

Their head and neck should be in neutral alignment, as should their TPC (as described in the earlier patterns). Some individuals will need to have their legs anchored so that they can create flexion of the trunk and spine without their legs lifting off the surface. However, try not to allow the individual to over-rely on this stabilization: if they need excessive anchoring to perform the movement, then use the regression pattern described below.

- The individual begins by gently flexing their head and neck by tucking their chin toward their chest and while segmentally flexing—flex one segment, followed by the next, etc.—their spine. It is important that the individual initially moves slowly, so that they can feel and develop control of the flexion through the neck, thorax, and lumbar spine.
- Once they have moved through thoracic and lumbar spine flexion, they anteriorly rotate their pelvis to continue the forward bending movement.
- When they have achieved as much motion as they can without forcing their body into the end range, the individual reverses the movement by first posteriorly rotating their pelvis, and then segmentally extending the lumbar, thoracic, and cervical spines. This is continued until they return to the starting position, with the TPC in neutral alignment. Ensure that they eccentrically control this motion with their psoas and abdominals, and that they do not simply drop back down into the supine position.

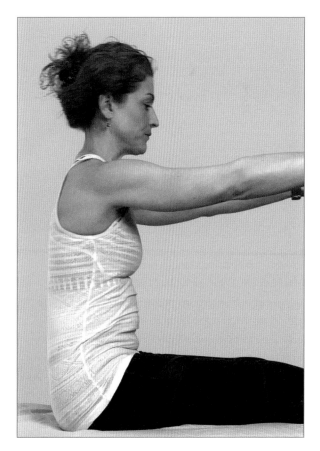

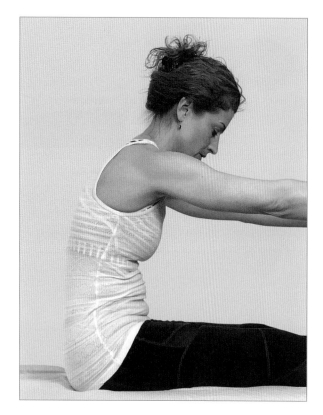

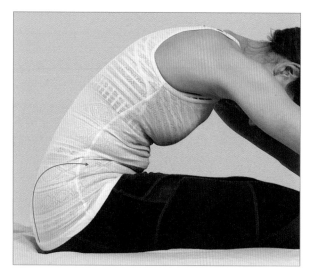

The Roll Up Pattern: The pelvis should continue to anteriorly tilt as the individual rolls up and forward (images above). Since the individual will compensate with excessive lumbar spine flexion, do not allow the individual to perform this pattern if they cannot keep their pelvis anteriorly rotating at the end of the pattern. As the individual rolls back to the table they will reverse the pattern beginning by posteriorly rotating the pelvis and segmentally extending the spine to return to the starting position.

For an additional challenge for those individuals that have demonstrated full range of motion through this pattern, the individual can hold a medicine ball or dumbbell in their hands for additional resistance during the pattern. Because of the risks involved with excessive loading and/or repetition of spinal flexion—especially in those individuals with a history of disc injury or other soft tissue/joint issue of the spine use caution when loading the Roll-up pattern.

Common Signs of Dysfunction in the Roll-up

The most common signs that indicate non-optimal psoas involvement during the Roll-up pattern are loss of segmental flexion of the lumbar spine and limited anterior pelvic rotation. It is not infrequent for individuals to have an inhibited psoas, and therefore does not contribute appropriately to segmental flexion of their spine. Similarly to the forward bending patterns described earlier, the loss of stability in the lumbar spine and pelvis-hip complex, and/or the lack of appropriate length in the glutes, hamstrings, and posterior hip complex, will limit one's ability to achieve a fully anteriorly rotated pelvis. These individuals will compensate for this lack of motion in one of three ways:

- by over-flexing through the thoracic and/or lower lumbar spine as they begin rolling up;
- by over-activating their abdominal wall, and posteriorly rotating their pelvis, while flattening (flexing) their spine onto the surface;
- by remaining in posterior pelvic rotation (tilt), rather than anteriorly rotating their pelvis as they get close to the end of the pattern.

Corrective Exercise Strategies for Improving the Roll-up Pattern

- *Release and/or lengthen myofascial restrictions.* Self-myofascial release, manual therapy release, and similar release strategies can be effective in releasing the restrictions in the erector spinae (especially around the TLJ) and in the posterior hip complex that are inhibiting the individual's ability to segmentally flex their spine and anteriorly rotate their pelvis.

- *Improve the function of the psoas in creating segmental movement of the spine.* The Articulating Bridge pattern (i.e. Pelvic Tilt pattern—see Chapter 2) is a much easier and lighter-loaded pattern to begin teaching/ training the concept of segmental spinal movement and rotation of the pelvis. Once the client has learned this movement through the Bridge pattern, use similar cues to help them create more optimal movement in the Roll-up pattern.

- *Limit the range of motion and/or use assistance.* Have the individual perform the pattern by just beginning to flex the head, neck, and upper thorax instead of trying to move through the entire spine. Have them hold a resistance tube or cable out in front of them, so that they use their arms to relieve some of their body weight, which will help with the lift. A way of using gravity to assist the movement as the individual develops coordination in the pattern is to start with their head and TPC slightly elevated relative to their legs (e.g. on a slight incline).

Side Bend

Setting Up the Side-bend Pattern

- The individual starts in the standing position, with their feet approximately shoulder width apart. The TPC is in neutral alignment and they should be supported on the feet tripods— most of the pressure will be under the first joint (or big-toe side of the foot), the fifth joint (or little-toe side of the foot), and the heel. The hip, knee, ankle, and foot should be aligned with each other, so that a straight line goes from the hip joint, through the middle of the knee joint, and to a point between the first and second digits of the foot.

- They visualize being long through their spine, and maintain this idea of length throughout the pattern. An excellent cue is to have them visualize a wire gently pulling them up and over a barrel that is placed by their side.

- After taking a deep breath into their hands, the individual breathes out while slowly side bending their trunk to one side, maintaining the length through their trunk and spine (arrow in image below right).

- The individual breathes in on returning to the starting position, and repeats the pattern to the opposite side. They should feel as if they are elongating their trunk and spine as they side bend, and attempt to maintain that length as they return to the starting position.

Because it tends to over-develop the quadratus lumborum and over-load the lumbar spine in a non-optimal manner performing resisted side-bending pattern is not recommended unless there is a specific sport or occupational requirement. Since many individuals generally have a hard time controlling neutral alignment let alone performing a pure side-bending motion with body weight. This

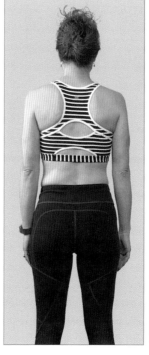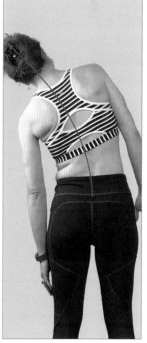

pattern is not generally performed with external loads. Because there are so many alternatives for training spinal motion, only when the individual has developed appropriate alignment and control of side-bending and there is a specific need, will they perform this type of pattern. Training control of side bending, see Carrying Patterns below, is a safer alternative for most individuals.

Common Signs of Dysfunction in the Side Bend

Similar to the Forward Bend, a common sign that indicates non-optimal psoas involvement and over-activity of the quadratus lumborum and/or

erector spinae during the Side Bend pattern is the loss of segmental motion. This results in a hinge, whereby there is preferential side bending through one region of the spine, rather than the use of the entire spine being contributing to the movement (image below right).

Corrective Exercise Strategies for Improving the Side-bend Pattern

- *Release and/or lengthen myofascial restrictions.* Self-myofascial release, manual therapy release, and similar release strategies can be effective in releasing the restrictions in the erector spinae and/or quadratus lumborum

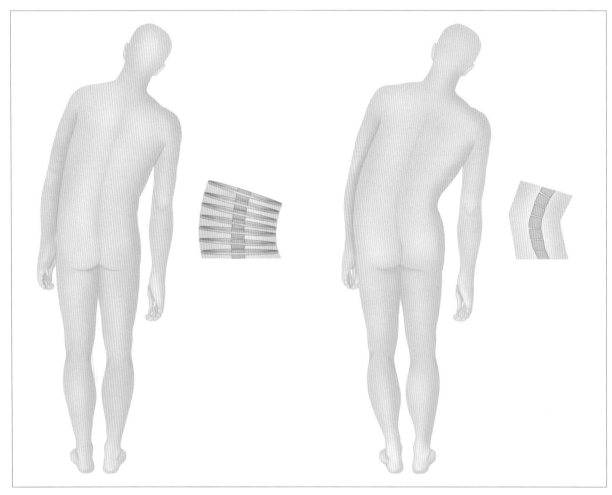

Side Bending: Optimal (left)—the entire spine elongates as the individual side-bends; Non-optimal (right)—the individual hinges or segmentally bends (laterally flexes) at one region of the spine rather than elongating and using the entire spine to contribute to the motion.

that are inhibiting the individual's ability to segmentally flex their spine.

- *Improve the function of the psoas in creating segmental movement of the spine.* The individual can visualize the TPC as an accordion or slinky that lengthens as it moves into side bending. Another option is to visualize the psoas on the side opposite the one they are bending toward (i.e. the right psoas if they are bending to the left), while keeping the vertebral segments connected. As they side bend, the psoas maintains the connection to the vertebral body as it lengthens. They can also visualize bending their trunk over the side of a barrel; this is useful for promoting length through the spine rather than hinging in one region. They can also imagine air pockets (or space) in between adjacent vertebrae, and try not to squeeze down on these as they side bend.
- *Use three-dimensional breathing.* The individual bends just to the point where they are restricted; they then take 1–3 breaths into that region, visualizing creating length or space between the segments, before returning to the starting position. As they gain the ability to lengthen with each set of breaths, they can bend a bit further, making sure that they are remaining long through their spine.

Carrying Patterns

While technically not a side-bending pattern, carrying patterns—also referred to as Farmer's Walk or Suitcase Carries—are great patterns for developing TPC (core) stability and strength (image right). Although they target the entire TPC, these patterns specifically train contralateral

(opposite side of the weight) stability of the core stabilizers-psoas, abdominals, erector spinae-in controlling potential side-bending of the spine that would result from the unilateral carrying position. Essentially this exercise becomes an anti-lateral flexion pattern. The pattern can be loaded with dumbbells, kettlebells, or other carrying device.

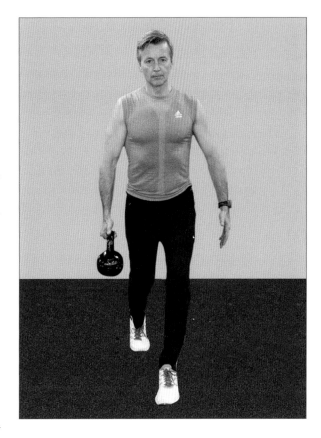

Unilateral Farmers Carry—As with most core patterns, the individual should maintain TPC alignment and remain long (suspended) through their trunk and spine. The weight should not cause the individual to compromise trunk, spine, or shoulder stability.

Summary of Psoas Function in Bending Patterns

At the trunk, spine, and pelvis

- Stabilizes the TLJ, lumbar spine, and pelvis to assist segmental motion of the spine in forward and side bending motions.
- Stabilizes the spine, pelvis, and hips to support anterior rotation of the pelvis over the femoral heads during both the Forward Bend and Hip Hinge patterns.
- Maintains neutral alignment of the lumbar spine and pelvis in the Hip Hinge pattern.

At the hip

- Acts as a functional synergist together with the gluteus maximus in centrating the femoral head within the acetabulum during the Forward Bend and Hip Hinge patterns.

Summary: Bending

1. During forward bending (forward flexion):
   - In standing, the psoas likely contributes to segmental flexion as the trunk and spine are flexed. In this role it is maintaining segmental control, so that forward bending is smooth and coordinated.
   - From the supine position, as in the Roll-up pattern, the psoas plays a more active role in segmental flexion of the lumbar spine, again assisting in smooth and coordinated movement.
   - In the Hip Hinge pattern, the psoas will help maintain neutral alignment of the TPC and hip centration as the pelvis rotates around the femoral heads.

2. During side bending (lateral flexion), the psoas may assist segmental side bending of the spine. The psoas on the side opposite to the side bending (i.e. the contralateral psoas) will eccentrically lengthen to limit and/or decelerate side bending of the spine.

3. During unilateral carrying patterns, the contralateral psoas and quadratus lumborum stabilize the spine to maintain an upright position.

Signs of non-optimal psoas function during bending patterns:

- Forward Bend: the individual remains in spinal extension (lordosis) and will not be able to segmentally flex their spine.
- Hip Hinge pattern: the lumbar spine flexes and/or the pelvis rotates posteriorly.
- Side Bend: the individual excessively side bends or hinges at one or two vertebral segments, rather than maintaining spinal elongation.

Spine and Hip Extension

Introduction

Another requirement in life is the ability to extend and resist the force of gravity that would otherwise pull us toward the ground. The extensor muscle groups of the spine and hips—erector spinae, glutes, and hamstrings—are often referred to as the *anti-gravity muscles*; as well as regulating internal pressure, these muscles are responsible for enabling us to maintain upright posture. Additionally, spinal extension allows one to reach overhead and bend backward in many of life's activities. Spinal extension also loads the anterior chain (pectoralis muscles, abdominals, psoas, and hip flexors) of the body, so that one can swing, throw, or launch an object, and perform many gym and recreational exercises.

"Elongation" and "lengthening" are two terms that will be frequently used in this chapter when discussing spinal extension. *Elongation* or *lengthening* refers to the ability to maintain joint centration and internal pressure regulation, so that the spine elongates or lengthens as one extends or backward bends. Optimal spinal elongation ensures that each segment of the spine contributes to extension, rather than just a single region being the primary area of motion.

It is the ability to suspend the thorax over the pelvis, regulate internal pressures, and maintain joint alignment and control that enables the erector spinae muscle group to extend the spine. Non-optimal joint alignment or control, pressure regulation, and/or over-compression by the myofascial system ultimately leads to compensatory motion during spine extension.

The ability to extend one's hips is a requirement for normal gait, including walking, running, and sprinting, as well as for other activities, such as skipping, hopping, and jumping. Many activities in life become compromised when one is not able to optimally extend their hips.

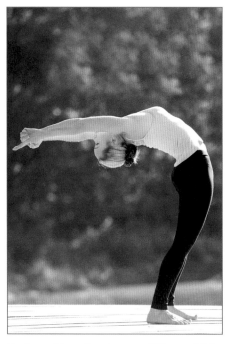 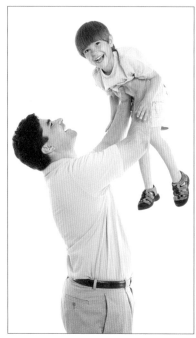 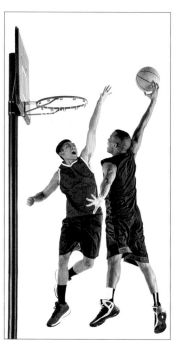

Backward bending in yoga, lifting a child overhead, and sports all require the ability to extend the spine and hips.

Psoas' Role in Spinal and Hip Extension

Optimal function of the psoas is required in order to safely and effectively perform both spinal and hip extension. To understand its' impact, it is important to understand what ideal motions should be occurring in these regions. When bending backward from an upright or standing position:

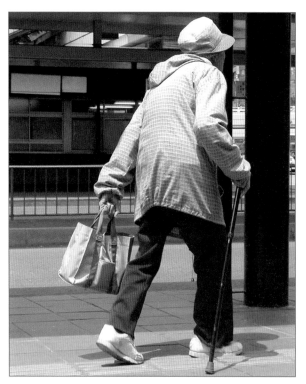

This woman is in posterior pelvic tilt and spinal flexion, a common posture in individuals with spinal stenosis, which limits her ability to fully extend her left hip. The loss of hip extension will require compensations through either the spine or lower extremity.

- the spine elongates and remains centrated as it extends;
- the pelvis posteriorly rotates over the femoral heads;
- the hips remain centrated.

The psoas is responsible for stabilizing the anterior aspect of the lower thoracic and lumbar spine, as well as for anchoring the pelvis so that the spine elongates during backward bending. When the psoas is unable to stabilize the spine and achieve spinal elongation, there will be over-compression of the posterior joints and soft tissue.

Commonly there will be a loss of ability to elongate the spine which results in compensatory hyperextension. As the individual extends or

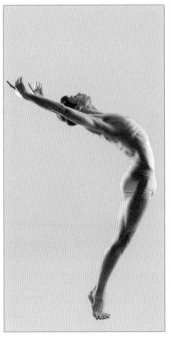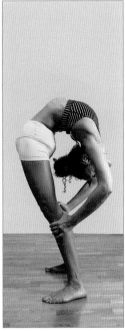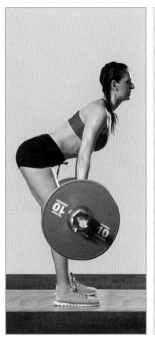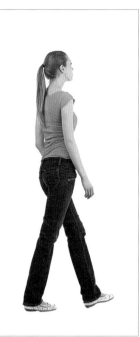

The dancer is able to maintain alignment of the thoracopelvic cylinder and lengthens his spine as he extends his hips and pelvis (left image). Example of extreme spinal extension in well-trained yoga practitioner (right image, supplied by, and copyright of, Alessandro Sigismondi. Model Laruga Glaser (larugayoga.com)).

The psoas helps maintain neutral alignment of the pelvis and spine when deadlifting (left image) and eccentrically lengthens to limit the amount of spine and hip extension as well as anterior pelvic rotation of the trail leg (right leg in right image) when walking.

bends backward, a "hinge" is created around the hypermobile segment(s) of the spine; this region of hypermobility will often be an area of discomfort and can contribute to early degenerative changes to of the spine.

The psoas also has a significant contribution to hip extension. Certain activities and exercises (for example when lifting out of a squat or deadlift pattern) require that the spine and pelvis either remain neutral (lumbar lordosis and anterior pelvic tilt) or extend back to neutral. The femoral head should remain centrated within the acetabulum as the hips are extended. In these situations the psoas works as a functional synergist together with the hip muscles in maintaining hip centration. The psoas also helps maintain alignment of the spine and pelvis during these patterns.

Activities such as walking, running and/or climbing a flight of stairs, however, require that

the pelvis anteriorly rotate on the side of hip extension. While an individual is walking, their psoas eccentrically lengthens to control excessive anterior pelvic rotation as well as the degree of hip extension. The psoas limits the amount of hip extension, thereby preventing anterior femoral head translation and excessive spinal extension, which in turn avoids over-compression of the lumbar spine. The following section will discuss strategies for improving elongation of the spine.

Prone Lengthen

As mentioned above, the ability to elongate or lengthen the spine is a prerequisite for optimal extension. Fittingly named by Sara Fisher, IMS™ (Integrative Movement Specialist™) and Jenice Mattek, LMT (Licensed Manual Therapist), IMS, Prone Lengthen is perhaps the most effective pattern for developing the ability to elongate the spine, as opposed to simply training spinal

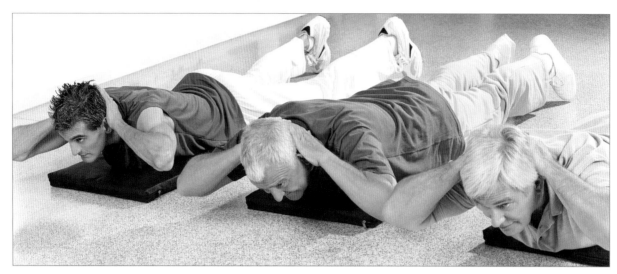

Individuals with limited ability to extend their spine will compensate by over-extending at their neck as noted in the image above, and/or thoracolumbar junction when performing back extension patterns.

extension. Prone Lengthen is a modification of the prone three month position used in Dynamic Neuromuscular Stabilization (Kolar et al. 2013). Additionally, the Prone Lengthen pattern is used to help individuals reinforce three-dimensional breathing; as well as lengthening the spine, it is one of the more effective strategies for actively decompressing the lumbar spine. Clinically, Prone Lengthen is one of the go-to patterns for individuals experiencing lumbar disc pain and radicular symptoms down the leg.

Why would one use the Prone Lengthen pattern and not simply use common exercises such as Superman and Hyperextensions to improve spinal extension? An explanation of this is warranted before discussing the details of the Prone Lengthen pattern. There are several problems with these exercises; in particular, they have a tendency to:

- teach spinal extension without a focus on elongation—especially in hyperkyphotic individuals, which leads to perpetuation of non-optimal spinal extension patterns;
- contribute to excessive hinging or segmental extension, generally around the thoracolumbar region, when there is an inability to lengthen the spine as the individual extends

(arrow pointing to hyperextension at the thoracolumbar junction image right);
- overdevelop the erector spinae and consequently over-compress the lower thoracic and lumbar spine, which, again, perpetuates a non-optimal backward bending strategy;
- overstretch and inhibit the psoas and abdominal wall, which contributes to the thorax being positioned behind the pelvis when in the upright position, further compromising both psoas and abdominal wall function;

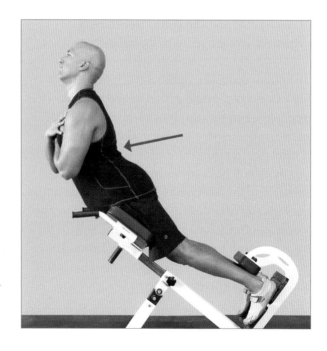

- be performed with too much resistance, too great a range of motion, and/or too rapidly, which hinders the individual from developing awareness and control of their thoracopelvic cylinder (TPC), in addition to overloading the lumbar spine.

Moreover, the overdevelopment of the erector spinae with the use of these exercises tends to inhibit the ability to breathe posteriorly. This limits the use of the posterior aspect of the diaphragm, leading to challenges in activating the deep myofascial system (DMS), and consequently negatively affecting both posture and movement (Osar 2015).

With an optimal TPC stabilization and extension strategy, however, there is no problem with individuals performing Superman and Hyperextensions provided that ideal form is used. The Prone Lengthen pattern can help individuals develop the awareness and control required to safely and effectively perform these exercises.

Setting Up the Prone Lengthen Pattern

- The individual begins by lying prone (face down) with their forearms in contact with the surface, their hands placed next to their ears, and their palms flat. Supporting their forehead on a towel or bolster will make this a relatively comfortable position (see image below). They will focus on keeping the lower portions of their anterior rib cage and pelvis in contact

with the surface. The ability to maintain this alignment throughout the pattern is an indication that the psoas and the DMS are appropriately maintaining positional control of the TPC.

A great cue to promote both optimal TPC and shoulder alignment is: "Stay open and wide through the front of your shoulders, and lengthen through the back of your head as if you are being gently pulled forward."

- The individual begins by breathing three-dimensionally, with the focus being on breathing inferiorly toward their pelvic floor and into their posterior rib cage. An effective cue to facilitate full expansion is to have them use their breath to fill their cylinder (the TPC) from top to bottom. As discussed in the breathing chapter (Chapter 2), do not allow them to force or rush their breath, and ensure that they are breathing in through the nose and out through their mouth.

Upon observation, their breath should gently cascade or move from their pelvis toward their head. Have them visualize a wire gently pulling them forward from the back of their head, and backward from their tailbone, to encourage lengthening of the spine (indicated by arrows in the images below). Perform 3–5 breaths in this manner for 3–5 sets.

- Once the individual has developed competence in this pattern, they should begin to gently lift their head off the support (image below). The individual lengthens their neck (arrow) as the head is supported off the table. They will inhale as described above and maintain length

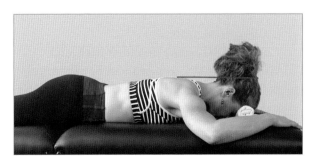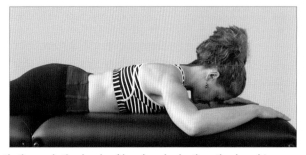

Prone Length—the individual maintains a sensation of length through the back of her head whether the head is supported (left) or lifting it off the support (right).

through the back of their head, neck, and upper thorax. They lower to the surface upon the exhalation.

To develop endurance of the DMS (deep neck flexors and multifidi) of the neck and upper thorax, the individual holds this position for several breaths, while continuing to focus upon maintaining length in their spine. They should work up to 3–5 breaths for 3–5 sets.

For demonstration of the Prone Length pattern, visit www.IIHFE.com/the-psoas-solution.

Common Signs of Dysfunction in the Prone Lengthen

There are three common signs that indicate non-optimal psoas involvement during the Prone Lengthen pattern:

1. *Non-optimal TPC alignment at the beginning.* Many individuals begin their pattern in thoracolumbar extension. There are several strategies to help restore optimal alignment:
   a. *Lengthen and decompress the thoracolumbar and lumbar regions of the spine.* If the practitioner is able to put their hands upon the client, gently traction each leg 2–3 times, alternating each side. The practitioner can also gently reach under the anterior rib cage and gently traction the front of the rib cage down toward the pelvis.

   If putting one's hands on the client is not an option, have them gently lengthen or reach each leg in an alternating fashion along the length of the table or floor. Performing this lengthening 2–3 times per leg will help lengthen their spine prior to beginning the Prone Lengthen pattern.
   b. *Release gripping in the thoracolumbar erector spinae muscles.* Use manual therapy and/or self-myofascial release to treat the hypertonic erector spinae muscles. The individual should breathe into the lower

posterior rib cage to facilitate release. Use the Happy Baby position with leg support, and perform 2–3 sets of three-dimensional breathing with a focus on using the breath to lengthen the TLJ prior to the prone position being assumed.
   c. *Cue connection to the psoas and abdominal wall.* Cuing can be very effective in establishing more ideal TPC alignment while in the prone position. Coordinate the following cues with three-dimensional breathing, selecting the one that resonates best with the individual:
      - Psoas cue: "Visualize a line from the front of your spine to the front of your pelvis, and maintain this connection as you lengthen from the back of your head as if you are gently being pulled forward."
      - Abdominal wall cue: "Imagine a line connecting the front of your rib cage to the front of your pelvis, and maintain this connection as you lengthen from the back of your head as if you are gently being pulled forward."
      - Pelvis cue: "Keeping your pelvis heavy upon the table, imagine a wire attached to your tailbone gently pulling your pelvis toward your feet, and lengthen from the back of your head as if you are gently being pulled forward."

2. *Excessive use of spinal extension.* Many individuals will rely solely upon their erector spinae muscles to lift themselves up, instead of elongating or lengthening their spine. This overactivity is often the result of overusing extension-biased exercises such as Superman and Hyperextensions.

Cue them to breathe into their back, and visualize the TPC as a cylinder or cylindrical ball filling up, rather than lifting themselves up using their back muscles. Have them shorten the range of motion, and focus primarily on lifting and lengthening through the back of their head, neck, and upper thorax, instead of actually lifting up toward the ceiling. It can be helpful to place one's fingers on the back of the client's head, so that they can kinesthetically recognize or feel that they are lengthening or reaching toward the practitioner's hand.

3. *Head and/or neck extension.* It is common to see individuals merely extending at the suboccipital and/or cervical spines, instead of lengthening through their spine. Use similar cues for lengthening discussed above, and shorten the range of motion while they focus on their breath in order to lengthen, rather than trying to lift their head off the towel support.

Backward Bend

The Backward Bend is not technically an exercise pattern, but rather a way to train a functional pattern required for daily life. This pattern will help the individual use their entire spine for overhead reaching, lifting, and/or backward bending, while minimizing the effects of spinal compression.

The Prone Lengthen pattern helps set up optimal spinal extension, because it teaches the individual how to elongate or lengthen their spine, instead of simply performing a backward bending motion. As mentioned in the introduction to this chapter, the inability to elongate the spine will lead to over-compression of the spine and generally a compensatory hypermobile region or spinal "hinge."

Setting Up the Backward Bend Pattern

- The individual begins in neutral alignment, standing with their feet together and arms at their sides.
- They begin by inhaling three-dimensionally. As they exhale, they slowly begin segmentally extending their head and neck, followed by their upper, mid, and lower thorax, as if they

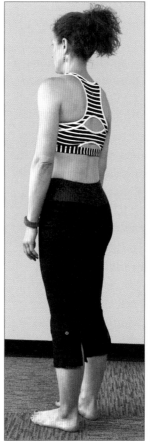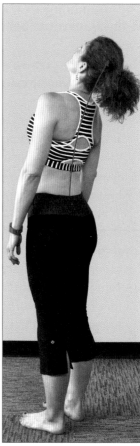

The client maintains length through her spine as she bends backward.

are gently being pulled toward the ceiling as they extend their spine (images above).

- If the individual's range of motion permits, they continue to extend through their lumbar spine and posteriorly rotate their pelvis over their femoral heads. There should not be excessive muscle activity in either their erector spinae or their glutes.
- Upon the next inhalation, they segmentally reverse this motion and return to the starting position.

When the Backward Bend is properly performed, there should be a smooth, coordinated curving of the individual's spine, and the individual will not report any feelings of posterior spine compression.

Common Signs of Dysfunction in the Backward Bend

There are two common signs that indicate non-optimal psoas involvement during the Backward Bend pattern:

1. *Excessive thoracolumbar extension.* When there is an inability to elongate or lengthen the spine, the individual can easily overextend or hinge at a particular segment of their spine. While this compensatory hinge can occur at any level of the spine, the TLJ will be the most common region. The issue generally occurs because either the individual is not appropriately elongating their spine, or they may be excessively kyphotic in the thoracic spine, which limits the contribution of this part of the spine to the motion.
   If they are not elongating their spine, cue them to connect to their psoas, and/or to lengthen through the back of their spine as they are extending. Have them use their breath to fill their TPC from top to bottom in order to assist elongation as they are extending. Their range of motion may also need to be limited until they develop the control required for greater ranges of motion. It is often better to work through ranges of motion that the individual can control than to force them through greater ranges that cause them to compensate.
   If the individual is hyperkyphotic in their thoracic spine, do not force the extension motion or they will simply over-compress their spine in the region in which extension is already taking place. Forcing spinal extension will rarely improve this range of motion in a hyperkyphotic individual; instead, try spinal mobilizations using Cat/Camel exercises or self-myofascial release prior to the pattern. Then have them focus more on the Prone Lengthen pattern until they have developed greater thoracic mobility in order to achieve thoracic spine extension.

2. *Anterior pelvic rotation with posterior translation of the thorax.* Rather than extending their spine, some individuals will simply anteriorly rotate their pelvis as they extend their thorax. Cue these individuals to maintain their TPC alignment and lengthen toward the ceiling as they extend. Have them place their thumbs on the lower aspects of their anterior rib cage and their fingers upon their anterior superior iliac spines (ASISs), so that they can monitor for the maintenance of this connection as they extend their spine.

Hip Hinge Bridge

Bridge patterns are one of the most commonly performed exercises in the rehabilitation and training industries. Some versions of this exercise make it into almost every rehabilitation program that targets low back or hip dysfunction, and nearly every program that targets the gluteus maximus has some iteration of the pattern.

Psoas' Role in the Hip Hinge Bridge Pattern

We discussed the Articulating Bridge pattern in Chapter 2. This section will focus on the Hip Hinge version of the Bridge pattern. In the Hip Hinge Bridge pattern the psoas takes on two primary roles:

1. Stabilization of the lumbar spine and pelvis.
2. Centration of the femoral head to ensure pure hip extension.

The Bridge pattern is commonly used to improve hip extension, which is also one of the benefits of the Hip Hinge version. However, the Bridge pattern should primarily be used for improving the ability to maintain neutral pelvic alignment throughout a relatively controlled range of motion. Too often, the individual is cued to squeeze their glutes as hard as possible, and lift the pelvis as high as possible. There are three problems with this:

1. Over-contraction of the glutes causes posterior rotation of the pelvis.
2. Too much activity in the glutes drives the femoral heads forward within the acetabula.
3. Posterior rotation of the pelvis leads to over-flexion of the lumbar spine.

This common strategy inhibits optimal use of the psoas and glutes; and has very limited applicability in encouraging proper use of the psoas and glutes while in the upright position.

The Hip Hinge Bridge was developed as a way of helping patients achieve more optimal co-activation between their psoas and gluteus maximus, while making sure that they remained in neutral TPC alignment throughout the pattern. When performing the Hip Hinge Bridge pattern, the goals are:

1. To activate the gluteus maximus, but without cuing overactivity in this muscle.
2. To maintain neutral alignment (slight anterior pelvic tilt) of the pelvis.
3. To ensure that movement only occurs through the hip joints during the pattern.

Setting Up the Hip Hinge Bridge Pattern

- The individual lies supine, with their elbows, hips, and knees flexed. Their hips, knees, ankles, and feet should be in a straight line and about hip-width apart. Their TPC should be aligned, and there should be neutral curvature in the spine. A small support can be placed under their head, so that it is also aligned; however, ensure that their head is not lifted too high, as motion of their body during the pattern can create excessive neck flexion.
- The individual begins by taking a few three-dimensional breaths. Upon inhaling, they lift up their pelvis and hold it elevated off the floor for 1–2 seconds. Generally, the individual is cued to lift their pelvis toward their feet. They should lift as high as possible, as long as they are able to maintain relative neutral alignment of the pelvis and spine. Recall that the goal of this pattern is to train pure hip flexion and extension, and not posterior pelvic rotation or spinal motion. The arms can be held off the floor to increase the challenge.
- The individual returns their pelvis to the floor, with no change in their alignment throughout the pattern. This means that their pelvis should still be in a slight anterior pelvic tilt, once they have lowered their pelvis.

If the glutes are used properly, there should be fullness in the posterior hip region. When they are over-gripped, a significant hollowing is created, which can be palpated in the lateral hip region. If the individual is comfortable with it, instruct them as to what proper gluteal activation feels

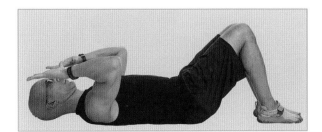 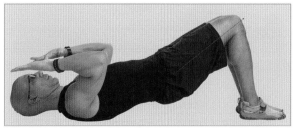

Hip Hinge Bridge—set up (left image); the individual is cued to maintain TPC alignment and lift their pelvis toward their feet (right image).

like, and have them palpate their own glutes, as this will be an important tactile cue for them to know, when they are performing the pattern on their own.

Common Signs of Dysfunction in the Hip Hinge Bridge

There are three common signs that indicate non-optimal psoas involvement during the Hip Hinge Bridge pattern:

1. *Non-optimal TPC alignment at the beginning, and/or lifting into excessive thoracolumbar extension.* Many individuals begin the pattern in thoracolumbar extension and/or non-optimal thoracic alignment (either too kyphotic or too lordotic). Prior to this pattern, have them perform three-dimensional breathing in the supported Happy Baby position to align their TPC. Note the thoracolumbar extension (arrow) when the individual is overusing their thoracic erectors and lifting the rib cage towards the ceiling (image below).
   Cue them to place their thumbs over the anterior aspects of their rib cage, and their fingers upon their ASISs, and ensure they maintain this distance throughout the pattern. Have them lift only as far as they are able to maintain this TPC alignment.

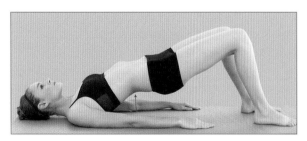

Thoracolumbar extension during the Hip Hinge Bridge.

2. *Posteriorly rotating the pelvis and/or flexing the lumbar spine.* This commonly occurs because the individual has prior experience performing the pattern in this manner. Instruct them that the pattern will be performed in a slightly different way, without any rotation of the pelvis or motion of the spine throughout. If the practitioner is able to place their hands upon the client, gently hold and guide their pelvis throughout the pattern, so that they get a sense of how to lift and lower it without creating posterior rotation.

3. *Anterior translation of the femoral heads through over-activating the glutes.* This is often another carry-over from previous performances of the pattern by the individual, during which they were cued to "squeeze" or "tighten" their gluteus maximus. Cue them to soften their activity and focus more on lifting their pelvis. Additionally, instruct them to lift as much as possible, but without squeezing or experiencing any change in their hip or pelvic alignment.

Marching Bridge and Single-leg Hip Hinge Bridge

Once the individual has mastered the double-leg version of the Hip Hinge Bridge pattern, they can progress to the Marching Bridge and Single-leg Hip Hinge Bridge patterns, which increase the demands of the glutes in controlling both hip extension and rotation of the pelvis (image below).

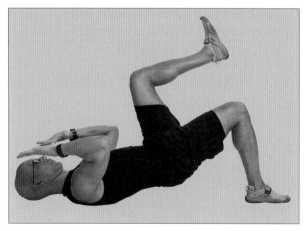

Marching and Single Leg Bridge Progressions—the individual maintains TPC alignment as they go through marching variations of the pattern.

Ensure that motion of the TPC is minimal, or zero, during the Marching Bridge, and that the pelvis remains level during both versions of the pattern.

For demonstration of the Hip Hinge and Marching Bridge patterns, visit www.IIHFE.com/the-psoas-solution.

Hip Thruster

Recently, the Hip Thruster pattern—a version of the Bridge pattern in which a barbell is placed over the pelvis, and the pelvis is "thrust" upward—has found its way into most strength and conditioning programs (image below).

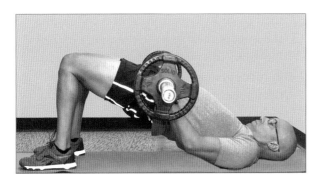

The use of this pattern has been ushered in as one of the go-to exercises for gluteal and *posterior chain* (posterior musculature of the body, including the calves, glutes, hamstrings, and spinal erectors) development. While glute involvement during the pattern cannot be argued, what is most concerning is the impact it has upon hip function.

There are several problems with this exercise as performed by the majority of patients and athletes that are clinically evaluated for hip and/or low back issues:

1. *Over-activation or excessive gripping of the glutes and posterior hip musculature.* This primarily results from using excessive loads during the pattern as well as from being cued to "squeeze the glutes as hard as possible," leading to hypertonicity of the glutes and posterior hip complex, over-compression of

the hip joint and ultimately to difficulty with hip dissociation.

2. *Anterior femoral head position.* This is due to over-activation or excessive gripping of the posterior hip complex as noted above. Over time, the excessive anterior hip position—also perpetuated by hip gripping during Squats, Deadlifts, and similar types of hip pattern—is a common contributor to impingement issues (see FAI in Addendum), labral tears of the hip, and other degenerative hip pathologies.

3. *Posterior pelvic tilt and resultant lumbar spine flexion.* This is also related to over-activation of the glutes and posterior hip complex and can potentially lead to lumbar disc and other spinal and pelvic pathologies.

As with most exercises, there is nothing wrong with performing Hip Thrusters if the individual performs the pattern with optimal mechanics. For general population clients and patients, the Single-leg Hip Hinge Bridge progressions discussed above adequately challenge the glutes and posterior chain.

To promote optimal mechanics during the Hip Thruster pattern, ensure that the individual maintains relative TPC alignment; make sure that they do not compromise their alignment by over-gripping the posterior hip musculature, tuck their pelvis into posterior tilt, pull their lumbar spine into flexion, and/or drive their femoral head excessively forward within the acetabulum.

Bird-Dog

The Bird-Dog pattern is another common rehabilitation and corrective exercise utilized to improve core stabilization and hip extension. Although considered an easy pattern to perform, technically it is highly challenging to perform correctly. Too often, the focus of the pattern is more on the motion of the arms and legs, rather than on coordinating synergistic activity between the elements of the core and ensuring optimal hip motion. Instead of benefiting the individual, the

Bird-Dog pattern frequently contributes to non-optimal core stabilization and hip extension patterns.

It is crucial to ensure proper form and execution of the Bird-Dog in order to derive the benefits and to minimize compensations during the pattern. The description that follows will only discuss movement of the leg, since many individuals will struggle to maintain lumbar spine control during the pattern.

Psoas' Role in the Bird-Dog Pattern

The psoas has two primary roles in the Bird-Dog pattern:

1. Stabilization of the lumbar spine and pelvis
2. Centration of the femoral head to ensure pure hip extension

Setting Up the Bird-Dog Pattern

- The individual assumes the quadruped position:
  - The TPC is neutral, and the head and neck are aligned relative to the TPC; neutral curves of the spine should be maintained.

- The hands are placed flat on the floor, just slightly forward and in line with the shoulders.
- The knees are directly under the hips and positioned just slightly less than hip-width apart; to maintain pelvic alignment the stationary leg is placed upon an elevated pad or surface.
- Because this is a challenging pattern, most individuals will begin with their knee flexed at 90° which reduces the moment arm prior to straightening their leg.
- In the quadruped position, the individual begins three-dimensional breathing to train coordination between breathing and isometric control of this position.
- From this position, the individual activates their psoas by visualizing a wire connecting the front of their spine to the center of their hip joint. This cue helps to activate the psoas in order to maintain isometric control of the lumbar spine and hip centration during extension.
- The individual slowly begins lifting their leg and then slowly lowers it repeating for the appropriate number of repetitions. There should be minimal to no motion of the trunk, spine, or pelvis as the leg is moved.

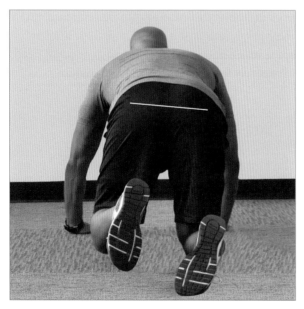 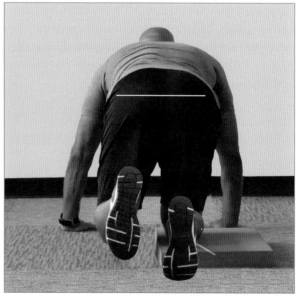

Many individuals will rotate their spine and unlevel their pelvis to clear the knee from the ground (image left).
Placing a support under the stationary leg helps to maintain neutral spinal and pelvic alignment (image right).

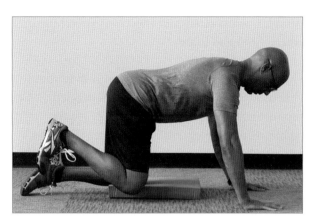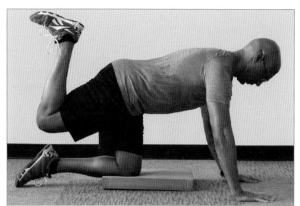

Modified Bird Dog—the individual extends their leg only as far as they can maintain neutral TPC alignment.

Note: To improve overall hip and TPC function, it is more important that they focus on controlling their position rather than how high they are actually lifting their leg.

- If the individual has trouble controlling their spine or pelvis, they can visualize a wire connecting the front of their spine to the center of their hip joint. This cue helps to activate the psoas and other deep stabilizers to maintain stabilization of the lumbar spine and pelvis as well as hip centration during hip extension.

The individual lifts their leg only as high as they are able to maintain alignment and control of their TPC. As they develop improved control in addition to length through their anterior hip, they can lift the leg higher.

Once the individual has demonstrated competence in this pattern, they can reach their leg longer and/or raise their opposite arm to further challenge TPC stability and hip extension.

For demonstration of the Bird-Dog pattern, visit www.IIHFE.com/the-psoas-solution.

Common Signs of Dysfunction in the Bird-Dog

There are three common signs indicating non-optimal psoas involvement during the Bird-Dog pattern:

1. *Non-optimal TPC alignment at the beginning.* Many individuals begin their pattern in thoracolumbar extension and/or non-optimal thoracic alignment (either too kyphotic or too lordotic). Reposition them into neutral TPC, and cue them: "Imagine a wire pulling you gently forward from the back of your head, and another one pulling your tailbone in the opposite direction." They should maintain three-dimensional breathing as these cues are given. Ensure that they are able to maintain this position for several sets of breathing, before allowing them to move their leg.

2. *Loss of neutral lumbar spine control as the leg is initially lifted.* It is especially important to note what happens as soon as the individual initiates movement to lift their leg. A subtle shift or rotation can frequently be observed in their lumbar spine as they transition their weight onto the support leg—this is a classic sign of non-optimal control. Cue them into using their psoas, and have them "visualize a wire connecting from the front of their spine to their anterior hip" before just initiating the act of lifting their leg. They must be able to transition their weight onto their arms and support leg, with no change in their spinal position as the leg is raised.

3. *Excessive anterior pelvic tilt and/or thoracolumbar extension, rather than pure hip extension.* These issues are usually related to a loss of lumbar spine control, as mentioned above and/or the inability to dissociate the hip. For those with lumbar spine control issues,

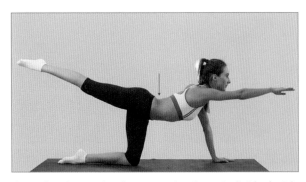

Excessive thoracolumbar extension in an individual with non-optimal psoas and core control.

cue the individual to activate their psoas, transversus abdominis and/or pelvic floor prior to initiating the leg lift.

Many individuals are unable to optimally dissociate or move the femoral head independent of their pelvis. In these circumstances, the lack of hip dissociation causes the entire pelvis or lumbar spine to move as the leg is lifted. For some, this issue is simply related to myofascial restrictions around the hip, in which case release the restrictions and repeat the pattern. For others, it is a motor control issue—they do not have a great strategy for moving the leg while controlling motion of their pelvis and spine; in this situation, the Side Lying Iso Hip Extension pattern is a great way to train TPC control with hip extension prior to performing the Bird-Dog pattern.

Side Lying Iso Hip Extension

While not a traditional psoas exercise, the Side Lying Iso Hip Extension (SLIHE) pattern is one of the best ways to train activation of the glute

complex, while safely and effectively stretching the anterior hip and thigh.

This pattern was designed as a way to train the gluteus medius in individuals who struggled supporting themselves while in single leg stance (standing on one leg). Although decent patterns for training hip dissociation in the early phases of hip rehabilitation existed, there were several limitations noted in many individuals during traditional Clam Shell and Side Lying Hip Abduction exercises:

1. While the Clam Shell and Side Lying Hip Abduction exercises were designed to improve gluteus medius strength, many individuals did not demonstrate improved strength, either in isolated muscle tests or in the single-leg test, even after performing the exercises for several weeks.
2. Most individuals were performing these exercises rather mindlessly; in other words, they could do 30, 40, 50, or more repetitions of the Clam Shell exercise and abduct their hip through significant ranges of motion without paying much attention to the movement itself. They were often compensating by rotating or side bending their spine and pelvis, rather than actually moving their hip joint.
3. There was not much functional carry-over from these exercises to the upright position and to single-leg standing.

The SLIHE pattern was created because of the limitations of these traditional rehabilitation exercises. After experimenting with the SLIHE pattern more in the clinic, patients and clients expressed positive feedback on how their hips felt after performing it. Moreover, they began

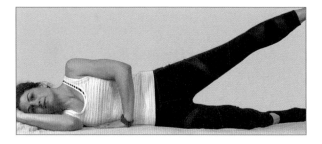

Clam Shells (left); Side Lying Hip Abduction (right).

demonstrating positive objective gains, including increases in isolated hip strength and range of motion. More astounding was that these changes were almost immediate, and there seemed to be a significant carry-over to upright single-leg stability.

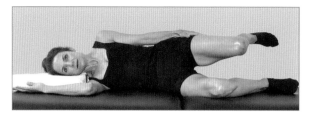

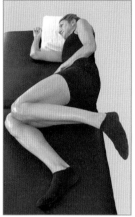 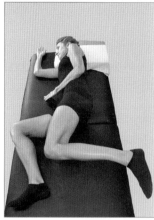

There are three primary benefits of the SLIHE pattern:

1. It trains isometric co-activation of the psoas and entire gluteal complex, rather than just the hip abductors and/or rotators.
2. It lengthens the superficial hip flexors as well as the fascia of the hip and thigh, without inhibiting the psoas; inhibition of the psoas is common in traditional versions of anterior hip stretches.
3. It trains the entire body, including ipsilateral (same side) stabilization of the shoulder and TPC, and the hip complex on the supported side (side they are lying on).

These benefits make the SLIHE pattern truly one of the most beneficial corrective exercise patterns clinically used to improve overall hip function. The biggest challenge with the SLIHE pattern lies in the set-up; therefore take an extra few moments to ensure that the individual is set up properly in order to achieve the maximum benefits from this pattern.

Setting Up the SLIHE Pattern

- The individual lies on a table on their side, with their spine and pelvis flat against a wall; their head should be supported so that it is aligned with their body. Their shoulders and legs should be stacked, with 90° of elbow and shoulder flexion, ~60° of hip flexion, and 90° of knee flexion. Essentially, they should be in neutral alignment when they are properly positioned (images above right).
- The individual begins by gently pushing their supported elbow and knee into the table—this should be only about a 10% effort. By isometrically pressing into the table, they are activating both the shoulder and

The Side Lying Iso Extension pattern—(front view, top image); basic set up (bottom left image); progression, moving the body further from the wall (bottom right image).

the hip stabilizers as well as the ipsilateral TPC muscles. This action should create a lengthening through their spine, and their rib cage should lift slightly off the table.

- The individual then raises their top leg so that it is in line with their body, and places their foot flat against the wall. Bare feet are usually easier to support on the wall than stocking feet. Holding their foot flat against the wall, they push isometrically into the wall with no more than 25% of their maximum effort. The goal is to activate the hip abductors and extensors on this side, with no change in the set-up position. The individual holds this position for 5–10 seconds and rests, before repeating for the desired number of repetitions. Generally, the individual performs 3 sets of 5 repetitions per side, with holds of 5–10 seconds per repetition.

For demonstration of the SLIHE, visit www.IIHFE.com/the-psoas-solution.

To progress this pattern, the individual moves away from the wall (image above right). Ensure that they are still stacked and aligned as in their original position against the wall. The further away from the wall they move, the more they will be actively lengthening the superficial hip flexors and the anterior hip and thigh fascia. Be sure to use previous psoas cues to keep them aligned and controlled throughout the pattern.

Common Signs of Dysfunction in the SLIHE

There are two common signs that indicate non-optimal psoas involvement during the SLIHE pattern:

1. *Non-optimal TPC alignment at the beginning.* Some individuals begin the pattern out of neutral alignment. The most common issue is that they do not have their shoulders or pelvis stacked—their bottom, or supporting shoulder and/or hip will often be forward, and so they will be leaning against the wall rather than being in a stacked position. Have them sit up and reposition themselves, ensuring that their shoulders and hips are stacked, and that their back is against the wall.

2. *Excessive anterior pelvic tilt or thoracolumbar extension, rather than pure hip extension.* Especially when the individual moves further away from the wall, they may not be connecting to their psoas and deep myofascial system (DMS), and thus may be losing TPC alignment as they engage their glutes. Cue them to connect to their psoas—"Visualize a wire connecting from the front of the spine to the anterior hip"—while engaging their glutes.

Clinical Considerations: 'Tight' Hip Flexors and Iliotibial Band Syndrome in the Active Population

In light of the discussion on tightness and stretching, many readers may be wondering about their clients or patients who exhibit chronic 'tightness' of their psoas. It is common that active individuals, especially runners, present with a self-diagnosis of a 'tight' psoas and 'weak' glutes.

Rarely is the individual actually accurate in their self-assessment of psoas tightness. Rather, virtually every individual that presents with chronic hip tightness points to the front of their thigh and more specifically, towards the attachments of their tensor fascia latae (anterior, lateral hip area) or their rectus femoris (anterior, superior region of the thigh). See left image opposite.

There are three situations that contribute to the sensation of anterior hip tightness:

1. The individual has shortened their superficial gluteus maximus and hamstrings and pulled themselves into posterior pelvic tilt thereby over-stretching their superficial hip flexors.

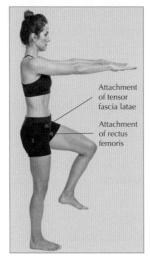
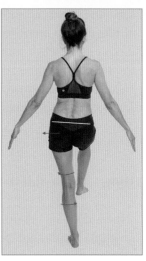

Attachment of tensor fascia latae

Attachment of rectus femoris

Attachments of the tensor fascia latae and rectus femoris (left image). Non-optimal control in single leg stance can contribute to overusing the tensor fascia latae and quadriceps when walking and during single leg exercises thereby causing the sensation of 'tight' hip flexors. Note the internal femoral rotation and external tibial rotation which occurs with non-optimal alignment and control of the pelvis and lower extremity (right image); this 'winding' of the lower extremity is a common cause of iliotibial band syndrome.

This gives them the sensation of 'tightness' in their anterior, lateral thigh region and hence, 'tight hip flexors.' To test this sensation, simply stand and place the fingers over the TFL and quads. Get a sense of the amount of tone in these muscles. Then tighten the glutes and hamstrings and pull the pelvis into posterior tilt. Note the increased tension and sensation of 'tightness' in the TFL and quadriceps. These muscles are now over-stretched and tight. Many individuals are living in posterior tilt of their pelvis and therefore will chronically feel as though they have 'tight' hip flexors when in actuality, their hip flexors and psoas are functionally over-lengthened.

2. The individual has an inhibited psoas and overuses their tensor fascia latae or rectus femoris in the role of hip flexion. Recall that both the tensor fascia latae (TFL) and rectus femoris have better mechanical advantage for hip flexion than the psoas (see functional anatomy in Chapter 1); however, they can become hypertonic and develop trigger points when overused. Generally, this is noted when performing a lying exercise with hip flexion like the Happy Baby with Heel Drops (pages 81–82) and excessive activation or even cramping occurs during hip flexion (concentric phase) or when lowering the leg from a hip flexed position (eccentric phase). Similarly with the Roll-up Pattern (pages 134–135) the individual may experience tightness or cramping in their TFL and/or rectus femoris as they anteriorly rotate their pelvis.

3. The individual has non-optimal control when walking or running and overuses their tensor fascia latae and quadriceps (rectus femoris, vastus lateralis, vastus medialis, and vastus intermedius) for single leg stability. This is also the most common cause of *iliotibial band syndrome*—tightness and irritation of the iliotibial band, secondary to non-optimal

alignment of the TPC and excessive internal rotation of the femur with external tibial rotation (see image p. 156 right).

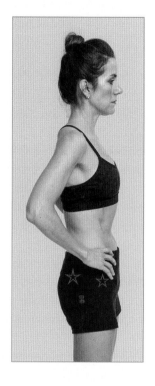

A quick and easy assessment to evaluate pelvic stability and muscle activation of the TFL and glutes is: The individual stands and places their fingers over the tensor fascia latae (TFL) and thumb over the gluteus medius (GMd) behind the greater trochanter (see 'stars' in image right). Then they raise the opposite leg and feel for pelvic position and contraction of the TFL and GMd under their fingers. With optimal co-activation of the TPC and hip stabilizers, there should be relative equal contribution between the TFL and GMd and the pelvis remains relatively level with minimal lateral tilt or rotation. In individuals with non-optimal TPC or hip control and/or chronic hip flexor tightness, it is common to note excessive TFL activation (the individual will feel a significant contraction of their TFL relative to their GMd) and the pelvis will either excessively laterally tilt or rotate.

The strategies presented in this book—specifically improving alignment and control of the TPC and hip while releasing excessive contraction of the glutes and posterior hip muscles—have been successful in helping individuals alleviate chronic hip tightness and restore efficient core and hip function. See more on this topic in Appendix I: Assessing the Psoas.

The individual may also be trying to overly muscle the pattern by pushing their foot into the wall with too much force. Have them use less force, and cue them to "engage the wall" with their foot, rather than trying to push their foot through the wall.

Stretching the Psoas

While there are countless articles, books, and videos about stretching the psoas—it would be remiss to not address this topic. Note: if the reader has had successful outcomes such as strengthening the psoas and glutes, decreasing low back or hip pain, etc. by stretching the psoas, then they are encouraged to continue using this strategy.

At Chicago Movement Specialists, stretching is rarely a part of the rehabilitation or training program for individuals experiencing low back and/or hip issues. There are several key reasons for this:

- Seldom is anterior hip tightness related to a short, tight, or overactive psoas. Moreover, if there is psoas overactivity and/or shortness, it is usually compensatory and protecting the lumbar spine; in these situations, stretching the psoas is generally not the best intervention option.
- There is too great a risk of overstretching and inhibiting the psoas using traditional stretches. Clinically muscle testing of the psoas and glutes is performed before and after a patient demonstrates what they have been doing to stretch their hips; almost 100% of the time, the stretch weakens (inhibits) both the psoas and the glutes. As a rule of thumb, any intervention—stretching, strengthening exercises, manual therapy, etc.—should never weaken or inhibit a muscle. If the individual tests weak after stretching there is an increased likelihood they will develop compensations if they do not re-stabilize the inhibited synergistic muscles.
- Most individuals are not stretching what is actually short, tight, and/or hypertonic.

The muscle that the majority of individuals point to when they complain of tight hips is either their tensor fasciae latae or their rectus femoris. Recall that both of these muscles are primary hip flexors, more so than the psoas. Often these two muscles become overactive and hence tight when they are overused as pelvic stabilizers. When the individual attempts to stretch their tight hip flexors, more often than not they are stretching their psoas rather than their rectus femoris and tensor fasciae latae. Generally, the superficial muscles – in this case the rectus femoris and tensor fascia latae – tend to be more resistant to stretching while the deeper muscles, psoas, tend to be more easily lengthened. Here is a simple explanation to help illustrate to patients how stretching is generally not very specific to the muscle they are attempting to lengthen:

Picture two pieces of resistance tubing—a high-resistance one (yellow tubing) representing the rectus femoris and tensor fasciae latae, and a low-resistance one (purple tubing) the psoas. When you individually stretch these two pieces of tubing (muscles), which one stretches first and further? Naturally, the low-resistance one, representing the psoas, stretches first and further (bottom image). This is often what is happening when one is stretching their hip flexors; the superficial hip flexors are not really lengthening while the psoas becomes over-lengthened.

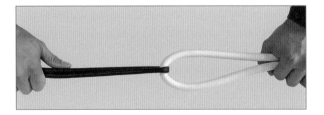

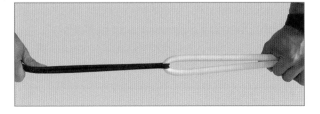

To counteract these effects, many trainers and practitioners will encourage their clients to pull their abdominals in and contract their gluteus maximus in order to stabilize the spine and pelvis as they perform the hip flexor stretch. Since so many individuals are already stuck in a posterior pelvic tilt and lumbar spine flexion, it is not advantageous to have them use this strategy, as it simply overstretches them further into this undesired position.

Manual therapy, Mindful Release™, and/or self-myofascial release work well in releasing hypertonicity in the superficial hip flexors. However, any manual release or self-myofascial release technique should always be followed up with a stabilization exercise. The Hip Hinge Bridge and Side Lying Iso Hip Extension patterns are great exercises to coordinate psoas and glute activation, while lengthening the muscles and fascia of the anterior hip and thigh.

Another effective lengthening technique for the superficial hip flexors is the Half-Kneeling Hip Stretch. While it technically looks like a traditional stretch, the pattern is really designed to lengthen the superficial hip flexors and anterior fascia, rather than simply attempting to stretch tight muscles. The important concept is that the pattern is performed with mindful attention to what is occurring, while resisting the temptation to obtain or "feel" a greater stretch in the hip flexors. It is important to not equate the sensation of feeling the stretch with the effectiveness of the pattern; indeed, it is more advantageous to experience less stretch and better overall centration, than to try to "feel" a more intense stretch.

Setting Up the Half-Kneeling Hip Stretch

- The individual aligns their TPC and half-kneels upon a stack of foam pads or towels. Their front hip and knee (non-kneeling side) are flexed to 90°.
  Since many individuals will not be able to achieve neutral pelvic alignment when placing

their knee on the floor, raising their bottom leg up will generally level and align their pelvis. Leveling the pelvis is a prerequisite for performing this pattern and ensuring optimal psoas involvement.

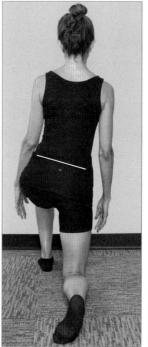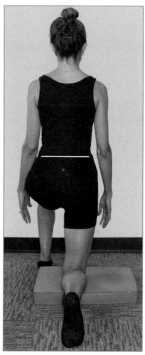

Half-Kneeling Hip Stretch—Many individuals will be unable to level their pelvis in the half-kneeling position (left image) and therefore will require support under their knee to level their pelvis (right image).

- Next, the individual cups their hand around their hip on the kneeling side, so that they can monitor the femoral head position. Being able to monitor the femoral head position when they are exercising on their own is an important point. Their thumb is placed behind the greater trochanter and their fingers are placed just medial to the ASIS.
- The individual is cued to connect to their psoas. The most consistently effective cue is: "Visualize a wire connecting from the anterior spine to the anterior hip, and maintain the length of this wire throughout the pattern."
- The individual then begins to shift their weight toward their forward leg. They are

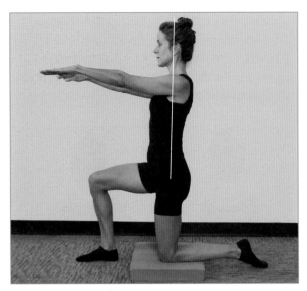 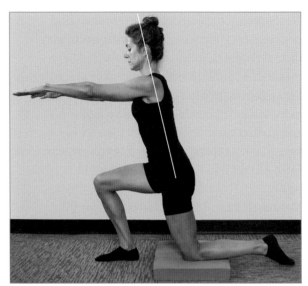

The individual aligns their TPC and maintains this alignment as they shift forward so they are able to lengthen the front of their hip. Note: the arms are held up so that the position of the pelvis and hip can be visualized.

monitoring that no bulging occurs under their fingers, or that there is no translation of the greater trochanter forward in front of their thumb. This ensures optimal centration of the femoral head within the acetabulum. Having them maintain joint centration with three-dimensional breathing is an incredibly effective strategy for improving both hip stabilization and tissue lengthening.

For demonstration of the Half-Kneeling Hip Stretch, visit www.IIHFE.com/the-psoas-solution.

Common Signs of Dysfunction in the Half-Kneeling Hip Stretch

There are three common signs that indicate non-optimal psoas involvement during the Half-Kneeling Hip Stretch:

1. *Beginning with non-optimal TPC alignment.* Some individuals begin the pattern out of neutral alignment. The most common issue is that they will not have their pelvis aligned and/or their thorax stacked over their pelvis. Have them stand up and reposition themselves, ensuring that their TPC is aligned and their pelvis is level, and kneel back onto the pads.

Some individuals will not have the flexibility to achieve flexion in the forward hip and therefore neutral alignment of the pelvis. Manual release and/or self-myofascial release can relieve the soft tissue restrictions in the posterior hip, enabling better hip flexion. As demonstrated on page 159, a support placed under their opposite knee is also helpful for aligning the pelvis.

2. *Anterior femoral head translation.* As discussed above, when stretching the hip flexors it is common for the femoral head to anteriorly migrate (excessively slide forward) within the acetabulum. If this motion of the femoral head is not controlled, the hip can become decentrated, and the psoas inhibited. Have the individual reset their position, and ensure that they are able to detect when the femoral head is anteriorly translating. Cue them to connect to their psoas as they lengthen their anterior hip, stopping as soon as anterior migration is felt under the fingers while the femoral head position is being monitored.

3. *Overextension at the TLJ.* This usually results from the individual trying to stretch too far, causing them to hyperextend at the TLJ. Cue the individual to connect their TPC, and maintain this alignment as they perform the

pattern. To monitor TPC alignment, have them place their thumbs over the lower anterior aspects of their rib cage, and their fingers upon their ASISs, and repeat the pattern.

The superficial hip flexors can also be performed in the split stance position to encourage lengthening through the anterior hip and thigh during hip extension patterns. Successful control of the spine, pelvis, and hips during this pattern is a prerequisite for performing many yoga poses, such as Warrior I. Be sure to encourage optimal TPC alignment, and monitor the femoral head position throughout the pattern. In the upright version:

- The individual begins by aligning their TPC and hips over their feet tripods.
- The individual activates their psoas, and moves one hip backward as far as they can, without the femoral head translating forward (they are monitoring the hip of their rear leg).

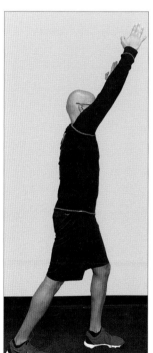 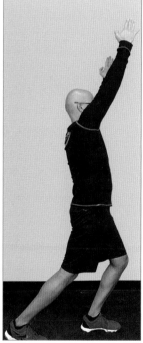

Standing hip flexor stretch with TPC controlled (left image) and not controlled (right image). Note the arms can be held overhead to increase the stretch on the anterior flexor chain.

- As previously described, at the point where they can no longer control the femoral head, they take a few three-dimensional breaths and visualize lengthening through their anterior hip and thigh. As they gain length, they will be able to gradually move their leg further behind them, to the next soft tissue barrier.

Summary of Psoas Function in Extension Patterns

At the trunk, spine, and pelvis
- Stabilizes the TLJ, lumbar spine, and pelvis to assist spine elongation during backward bending.
- Maintains neutral alignment of the lumbar spine and pelvis during hip extension.
- Eccentrically controls spine and pelvic alignment during backward bending and while walking.

At the hip
- Acts as a functional synergist together with the gluteus maximus in centrating the femoral head within the acetabulum during hip extension patterns.
- Helps controls excessive hip extension during common patterns, such as squats, lunges, and deadlifts.
- Eccentrically lengthens to control excessive hip extension during gait.

Summary: Spine and Hip Extension

1. During spinal extension (backward bending), the psoas stabilizes the spine and pelvis, thus preventing excessive joint and soft tissue compression. In particular, the psoas anchors the TLJ, lumbar spine, and pelvis to enable elongation as the spine is extended.

2. The psoas helps control the pelvis during backward bending, so that posterior rotation of the pelvis over the femoral heads is smooth and coordinated.

3. The psoas works with the lower fibers of the gluteus maximus to maintain femoral head centration within the acetabulum during hip extension. This enables the hips to remain centrated, which directly contributes to the ability to maintain the pelvis in a neutral (anterior pelvic tilt) and level position through hip extension patterns, including squats, lunges, and deadlifts.

Signs of non-optimal psoas function during hip extension patterns:
- Excessive anterior femoral head translation and/or excessive anterior pelvic rotation during movements or exercises requiring hip extension.
- Hollows observed or palpated in the lateral gluteal region, created by the anterior femoral head position, in an individual when standing and/or as they move into hip extension.
- Excessive thoracolumbar extension or lumbar spine hinging, and/or an inability to elongate the spine during back bending.

Conclusion

"The more we learn the more we realize how little we know."

R. Buckminster Fuller

In this book I have attempted to expand the conversation, taking the perspective that there are some things we know, or suspect to be true, about the psoas, and there are quite a few things we do not really know about it.

Here is what we know (or, more accurately, suspect) about the psoas at this time:

- The psoas has extensive attachments across the lower thoracic spine, lumbar spine, pelvis, and hip. It fascially blends into the diaphragm, transversus abdominis, quadratus lumborum, iliacus, and pelvic floor. These attachments suggest that the psoas has a much greater role than simply as a flexor of the hip and trunk.
- The psoas plays a role in unilateral hip flexion—as a stabilizer of the hip (helps centrate the femoral head within the acetabulum) on the side of hip flexion, as well as of the trunk and spine on the side opposite to hip flexion.
- The psoas is the only muscle located on the anterior surface of the lower thoracic and lumbar spines, suggesting that it is an important stabilizer of these spinal regions.

Along with the multifidi, it stabilizes the spine, thereby preventing excessive anterior translation of the lumbar vertebrae during loading, bending, and rotation. The muscle eccentrically lengthens to control excessive extension of the spine and hip, as well as anterior rotation of the pelvis.

- Because of its attachments to the pelvis and to the pelvic floor, the psoas does not have the capacity to anteriorly tilt the pelvis. When short, however, the muscle will increase lumbar lordosis.
- A prolonged seated posture, especially sitting in lumbar spine flexion and posterior pelvic tilt, will inhibit psoas activity and decrease its contribution to spinal and pelvic stability.
- Excessive flexion-biased exercises and over-bracing the abdominal wall will tend to shorten the abdominals, flex the lumbar spine, and posteriorly rotate the pelvis; this will additionally have an impact on the ability to optimally use the psoas.
- Thoracolumbar hyperextension—excessive extension at the junction of the thoracic and lumbar spine—will inhibit optimal expansion of the posterior aspect of the rib cage during breathing, which ultimately impacts psoas function. This posture and overuse of the thoracolumbar erector spinae muscles for

postural stability and during movement overstretches the psoas and abdominal wall, thereby inhibiting optimal use of the psoas, abdominals, diaphragm, and pelvic floor.

Are there many more questions to be answered? Of course, the answer to that rhetorical question is unequivocally—yes. This book has only scratched the surface in relation to what we will one day understand and the strategies we will employ to enhance posture and movement.

I took quite a few liberties discussing the psoas' function throughout certain movement patterns in the book, because, as acknowledged above, there is still much we do not know about the psoas' role in movement. The more we delve into an area, the more questions it seems arise. Some of the questions that have yet to be fully explored include:

- Is the psoas even a hip flexor, or is it merely functioning as a stabilizer of the hip joint during hip flexion?
- What is the psoas' role during breathing? Does it anchor the lumbar spine to prevent excessive spinal extension with motion of the diaphragm and pelvic floor, or does it play a more extensive role in the breathing process?
- Is the psoas' involvement in rotation of the spine significant, or is it simply stabilizing the spine and maintaining a central axis as the larger muscles rotate the trunk and spine?
- Since the psoas crosses the anterior surface of the sacrum and pelvis, how much is it involved in stabilization and mobility of the sacroiliac joints?
- The psoas seems to be active during the hip flexion phase of the gait cycle, to help centrate the hip and assist hip flexion; it also eccentrically lengthens during the hip extension phase to stabilize trunk, spine, and hip extension and to prevent excessive anterior pelvic tilt. What is the contralateral psoas doing on the stance leg during the same points in the gait cycle? Is it merely stabilizing that side of the trunk, spine, and pelvis-hip

complex? While the answer appears to be yes, more research needs to be done with regard to the psoas' involvement in gait.

The longer I am in practice and the more individuals I see, the less confident I am in the things I once believed to be true. I think that this plays a huge part in gaining more knowledge and clinical experience. You are able to help more individuals because you know so much more, and you have many more clinical experiences and strategies to rely upon; however, in the process, you also become less confident and question the reason(s) why certain strategies work, and why at other times they do not.

Future research and clinical experiences may disprove some of the things I have suggested in this book, just as so much of what I once learned seems to be contradicted on a nearly daily basis. However, we must never let our ego become so great, or must never become so overconfident in our current knowledge of what is right, that we lose sight of the bigger picture; nor must we try to lock every single patient or client we see into a single stereotype, so that we can create a neat little treatment/training formula that applies to everyone. Yes, there are commonalities in many of the individuals we work with. Regardless, each individual presents with their own history and their own set of habits (developed from compensations related to injuries, traumas, and surgeries, things they have learned, concepts of what optimal posture and movements are, etc.). They also have their own beliefs of what it will take to move into a better place or to accomplish their goals. Our job—rather, our *responsibility*—as health and fitness professionals is to meet each individual where they are at without judgment, and to help them develop the most appropriate plan using the best strategies that we know.

Serve your clients with confidence, integrity, and humility. And never stop learning.

Yours in health,
Evan Osar

Assessing the Psoas

- Psoas' role in lumbar spine and pelvic alignment
- Assessment of psoas and superficial hip flexors length in the Modified Thomas Test
- Manual muscle testing of the psoas

This appendix comprises modified and adapted text taken with permission from *Functional Anatomy of the Pilates Core* by Evan Osar and Marylee Bussard (2016).

A discussion about the psoas would not be complete without discussing the psoas' involvement in the hyperlordotic lumbar spine and anterior pelvic tilt posture. As discussed in the anatomy chapter (Chapter 1), the psoas does not have attachments to the pelvis in a location where it can contribute to an anterior pelvic tilt. While the psoas can pull the lumbar spine into an increased lordotic position, it rarely does so without the presence of other simultaneous compensatory changes in postural alignment.

So what gives many individuals the appearance of having an excessive anterior pelvic tilt and

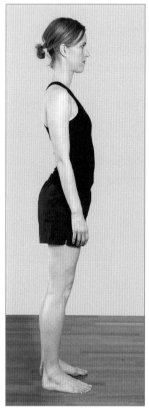 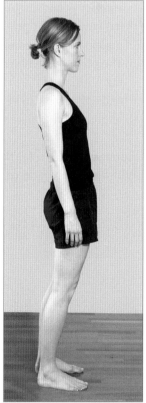

Thoracolumbar extension posture (left); sway back posture (right).

hyperlordotic lumbar curvature? There are two postural strategies that will contribute to these characteristics:

1. *Excessive extension at the thoracolumbar junction (TLJ).* This a common compensatory strategy for non-optimal core stabilization. It is also a strategy for making one's posture look more ideal, and often associated with postural cues such as "lift your chest up, and pull your shoulder blades down and back." This postural strategy makes it appear that the individual is in an anterior pelvic tilt, whereas the excessive extension is actually related to the posterior position of their thorax from over-activating the thoracic and lumbar erectors and from the relative overstretching of their psoas and abdominal wall. Often, when the thorax is properly stacked (aligned) back over the pelvis, the pelvic position is ideal.

2. *Sway back posture.* This is another posture that is often mistaken for lumbar hyperlordosis and an anterior pelvic tilt. In this posture the individual has swayed their pelvis forward, so that it is positioned forward relative to their trunk. The pelvis is often in a posterior tilt; however, the position of the pelvis relative to the trunk makes it appear to be in an anterior tilt, and the lumbar spine appear to be in hyperlordosis.

Common postures: (a) flat-back; (b) kypho-lordotic; (c)swayback; (d)kyphotic; (e) neutral.

Performing an accurate postural and length assessment is critical in evaluating the function of the psoas. See Appendix II for more details about neutral alignment and postural assessment.

Assessing the Length of the Psoas

The Modified Thomas Test is the gold standard for evaluating the length of the hip flexors, including the rectus femoris, tensor fasciae latae, and psoas. The test is performed by having the individual sit at the end of the table, pull one thigh into their chest, and lie back; the hanging leg is then evaluated.

Positive findings in the Thomas Test include:

- Psoas tightness if the thigh is held above the level of the table.
- Rectus femoris tightness if knee flexion is less than 90°.
- Tensor fasciae latae and iliotibial band tightness if the thigh abducts and the tibia is in external rotation.

However, myofascial tightness of the anterior thigh can create a false positive for psoas tightness during this test. Therefore, as part of

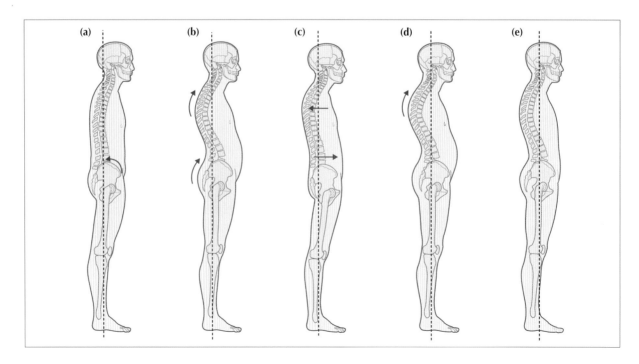

(a)   (b)   (c)   (d)   (e)

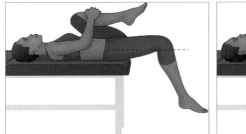 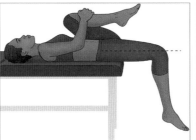 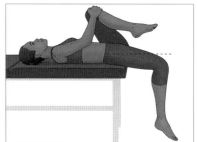

Modified Thomas Test: positive test (left image) for psoas shortness; negative test for psoas involvement (middle image); overlengthened psoas (right image).

the Integrative Movement System™ assessment process, it is only considered it true psoas involvement if the thigh is held above the level of the table *and* there is palpable hypertonicity (tautness) within the psoas muscle belly just superior and medial to the inguinal ligament (the angle of the psoas attachments along the spine). The presence of hypertonicity indicates that the muscle is truly contracted and shortened. On the other hand, if the thigh is above the height of the table and no palpable hypertonicity is felt in the psoas, the leg is being held up by myofascial tension in the anterior thigh, rather than being secondary to a short psoas.

Clinical example: this patient presented reporting low back discomfort and "core weakness." Her physical therapist had her stretching her psoas as part of her rehabilitation program, because she was assessed to be in an anterior pelvic tilt

and lumbar hyperlordosis. She was told this was causing her low back pain.

The patient was tested in the Modified Thomas Test—her psoas is actually overlengthened—her leg should be in line with her body, but is in fact lower. So what makes it appear that she is in an anterior pelvic tilt and lumbar hyperlordosis? In actuality, she is standing in thoracolumbar extension instead of having an increased lumbar lordosis; this is a common finding in individuals who have hip and low back issues. This issue is also related to the fact that she has well-developed glutes, and that the line of her pants exaggerates the visual appearance. Her psoas also tested weak (inhibited) on manual muscle testing. This patient is standing in thoracolumbar extension making it appear as if she is in an anterior pelvic tilt (left image); during the Thomas Test she demonstrates overlengthened psoas and hip flexors (right image).

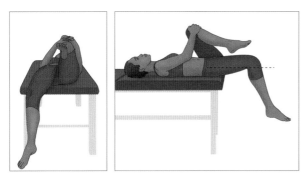

Shortness of the tensor fascia latae and iliotibial band—the leg should be in line with body rather than abducted (left image); shortness of the rectus femoris—the knee should be flexed at a right angle when at optimal length (right image).

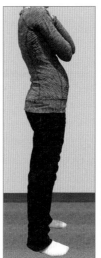 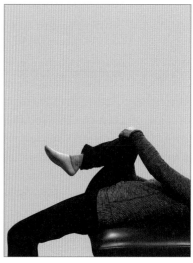

Muscle Testing the Psoas

This section contains modified and adapted text taken with permission from *Corrective Exercise Solutions to Common Hip and Shoulder Dysfunction* by Evan Osar (2012).

Manual muscle testing (MMT) can be utilized as an important evaluation tool in developing a corrective exercise, training, or therapeutic strategy (Osar 2012, 2015). While it is beyond the scope of this book to discuss all the nuances or the multitude of MMT methods, its use as an evaluation tool is unparalleled. Some question the validity, accuracy, and usefulness of muscle testing, but if performed properly, precision MMT can give the tester valuable information about the function of the client's nervous system and the integrity of their stabilization system.

Many readers are familiar with traditional MMT, which is taught in medical, chiropractic, and physical therapy schools. MMT as part of a functional assessment is demonstrated in the acclaimed book *Muscles: Testing and Function with Posture and Pain* (5th edition) by Florence Peterson Kendall et al. (2005). Traditional MMT as presented in this resource tests the specific strength of a muscle against an applied force. Increasing levels of force are used to overload a muscle and determine its overall strength; this is then graded on a scale of 0 (no muscle contraction at all) to 5 (ability to maintain muscle contraction and the test position against significant resistance).

MMT was later expanded upon by George Goodheart, DC through its use in Applied Kinesiology. Rather than testing the overall strength of a muscle, Dr. Goodheart used what would later be termed "muscle testing as functional neurology" to evaluate the efficiency of the nervous system in controlling the muscular system (Walther 2000). This muscle testing procedure did not test for strength or weakness, but rather how the muscle reacted to an applied force. Essentially, MMT as performed by Dr. Goodheart evaluated how the nervous system controls the myofascial system, and the response to the test can indicate when there is an underlying neuromuscular issue without evident pathology.

The late Alan Beardall, DC, a student of Goodheart, carried out further studies on the use of MMT; he was the first to demonstrate over three hundred muscle tests, one for each specific division of a muscle (Beardall 1982). Believing that muscles were the "display units of the body" (Buhler 2004), Beardall demonstrated that a muscle which initially tested strong could subsequently test weak if each division was tested individually. He went on to develop a system of evaluation and correction of this muscle inhibition, which eventually formed the basis of Clinical Kinesiology.

Additionally, Beardall pioneered testing each muscle division in its respective shortened position, or in positions that best approximated the origin and insertion. It was his opinion that the muscle mechanoreceptors were most sensitive in the lengthened position, and least sensitive in the shortened position (Buhler 2004). He therefore created a series of specific muscle tests to examine each individual muscle division in its shortened position.

Several of Goodheart's and Beardall's muscle testing concepts can be found in the following discussion of testing the psoas—specifically, the use of the shortened muscle position, the application of a 2-second constant resistance to the muscle (rather than steadily increasing resistance), and the interpretation of a muscle testing as either neurologically intact (strong) or neurologically inhibited (weak), versus grading a muscle test on a 5/5 type of scale.

A unique variation of the use of MMT is that of an overall evaluation of an individual's stabilization strategy (Osar 2015). When performing a MMT, there is less emphasis on the actual strength of the muscle, and more with the strategy the individual is using to stabilize their thoracopelvic cylinder (TPC) during the test. In other words, the strategy the individual is using to stabilize their trunk, spine, and pelvis is being evaluated during the muscle test. It is common to see improvements in TPC stabilization after performing an appropriate corrective exercise intervention.

Because of the depth of the psoas and the presence of other hip flexors, true isolation of the psoas is virtually impossible. Using the traditional muscle tests as described by Kendall et al. (2005), MMT of individuals who have had their psoas surgically detached still tested strong. In the test position, it is likely that these individuals are able to hold the position with their superficial hip flexors and adductors, even in the absence of an intact psoas muscle.

Although all muscle testing protocols obviously have limitations, the most clinically sensitive and reliable position to test the psoas, is posteriorly rotating the pelvis and adducting the thigh. In this position the other hip flexors and adductors

are placed at a disadvantage; therefore the psoas' function in maintaining the test position can be more accurately evaluated.

The following are contraindications to performing MMT:

- Acute low back, hip, or pelvic pain
- Labral tears of the hip
- Suspected tearing of the psoas, rectus femoris, or adductor muscles
- Hip replacement
- Cancer, vascular disease, or other systemic pathology

Psoas MMT Procedure

- The individual lies in a supine position, with their head straight, their arms at their sides, and their legs straight.

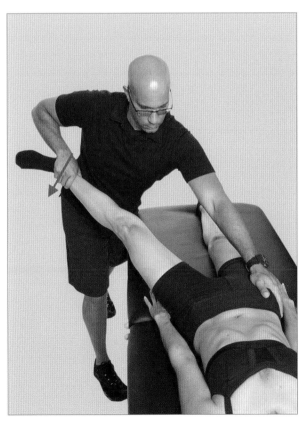 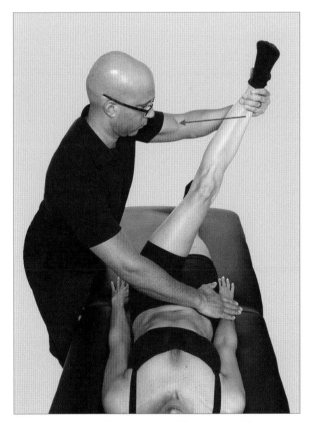

Psoas Manual Muscle Test—traditional psoas muscle test (left image); modified psoas test (right image)—this version tends to be more clinically sensitive to true psoas inhibition than the traditional version.

- With the knee straight, the tester fully externally rotates the hip and flexes the individual's leg, just to the point where the pelvis begins to posteriorly rotate, and then adducts the thigh just across the midline.

- The tester should keep his/her body near the test leg, in case the individual cannot hold the test position. Remember, with this type of muscle testing the goal is to test the individual's ability to hold the test position, rather than test the muscle's strength.

- The tester attempts to pull the individual's leg, and thus their pelvis, out of the test position for a two-second hold.

- A positive test is when the individual is unable to hold the test position, there is spasm in the adductors of the test leg, or pain occurs in the low back or groin area.

The length and strength of the psoas can be retested after myofascial restrictions around the trunk, pelvis, and hips have been released, a more ideal TPC alignment has been restored, and activation of the deep myofascial system has been improved using your corrective exercise strategy. Generally, with an improved TPC stabilization strategy, the muscle length and strength, and the overall ability to hold the test position, will be restored. Follow up any corrective exercise strategy by teaching the individual how to incorporate optimal use of their psoas into the appropriate functional exercises and activities. Several strategies for integrating the use of the psoas have been presented throughout this book.

For more information on the use of manual muscle testing, the reader is encouraged to investigate the resources given in the "Manual Muscle Testing" section of the Bibliography.

Neutral Alignment and Postural Assessment

Throughout this book the term "neutral alignment" has been used. *Neutral alignment* is a relative position in which the joints are optimally centrated (aligned and controlled) and the joint surfaces are in the most ideal positions to be loaded. Theoretically, when in neutral alignment, relatively little effort should be necessary for maintaining this position. Being out of neutral alignment therefore requires increased effort and energy expenditure to maintain this unaligned position. The more relatively aligned one's body position (i.e. neutral, or more optimal), the less the energy and effort required, and the less the potential wear and tear of the soft tissue and bony structures of the body.

Resources that refer to 'good' or 'ideal' posture are generally referring to a situation in which the

individual is in neutral alignment and using an appropriate strategy. For example:

"Good body posture is projected into the muscle tone (muscle balance or imbalance) and central control mechanisms, including psychological state, ligament conditions, and anatomical relationships are all reflected in posture. Posture also reflects reactions to pathological states within the organism." (p. 37, Kolar et al. 2013)

It is also important to note that neutral alignment is not meant to indicate that it should be a static, or non-moving, position. In actuality, the nervous system is continuously making micro-adjustments to one's position. It is the ability to make these micro-adjustments and move out of, and return to, a relatively neutral position that is a hallmark of a healthy and adaptable or robust system.

There are three primary characteristics of a healthy or robust postural strategy. These include:

1. the individual's postural strategy is relatively easy-to-maintain—during most activities of life it shouldn't require a lot of effort to maintain resting posture
2. the individual's postural strategy is adaptable—the individual can move into and out of a

variety of postures as required for their desired activities

3. the individual's postural strategy is sustainable—the individual can maintain their posture for long periods of time (years) without placing a significant amount of stress upon the soft tissue and/or bony structures (Osar 2015)

Generally, an optimal or healthy postural strategy supports a more optimal movement strategy and the movement strategy then reinforces more optimal posture. Conversely, the more compromised an individual's posture or movement strategy, the more they begin to perpetuate their habits. These non-optimal habits ultimately affect posture and movement and how they function. The three characteristics of a non-optimal postural strategy include:

1. The individual uses too much muscular effort to maintain their posture and thereby creates too much rigidity in their system; over time this tends to contribute to chronic myofascial tension and over-compression of joints which can lead to early degenerative joint changes.
2. The strategy is not readily adaptable meaning the individual tends to use a similar strategy for varying positions and activities; individuals with inefficient postural strategies tend to maintain relative static positions and essentially are 'locked' into a specific posture and then repeat this postural strategy for many activities of life; this can also perpetuate non-optimal movement habits and lead to early degenerative joint conditions.
3. The individual's strategy causes discomfort and/or places unwanted stress upon soft tissue and/or bony structures; again, potentially contributing to early degenerative joint conditions.

The goal of performing a postural assessment is never to 'correct', 'fix' or create 'perfect posture.' The primary goal of performing a postural strategy is first and foremost to identify the individual's current strategy for maintaining their posture and then determine if it is affecting and/or being affected by their movement strategy. Only when

their current strategy is causing discomfort or it is deemed to be affecting or affected by their movement strategy is posture itself addressed.

Postural Assessment

Postural assessment is an important part of the evaluation process, as it is the most accurate method for evaluating initial joint alignment and postural control.

While it should never constitute the only assessment performed, there are three primary benefits of assessing posture as part of a comprehensive evaluation process:

1. It provides a starting point for evaluating movement. Posture is the beginning and ending position of movement, and is a virtual snapshot of an individual's movement strategy. It is essentially how the nervous system coordinates muscle activity for stability when the body is in a static position. While not applicable to everyone, it is very common for an individual's postural alignment to reflect their movement strategy.
Another important component of analyzing posture is relating the individual's static alignment to their dynamic movement, and then determining whether or not what you note about their posture warrants greater attention or is worth addressing. For example, a client presents with low back tightness and weakness in hip flexion. During a postural assessment posterior pelvic tilt and lumbar spine flexion is observed; while this may not be an optimal static alignment, the clinician should determine whether or not this finding is driving or reacting to their primary issue. A very effective way to determine whether or not this issue should be addressed is to have the individual perform a more dynamic movement, such as a squat or a single-leg stance. If their alignment improves (i.e. they move into a more neutral pelvic alignment as they squat or stand on one leg, they align their

thoracopelvic cylinder (TPC) appropriately, and they are able to appropriately flex their hip without compensation), then it is probably not high on the priority list of things that need to be addressed. In this case it is likely that they have just learned a non-optimal postural strategy; however, it is not carrying over into their movement strategy. On the other hand, if they begin in a posterior pelvic tilt and it either persists or becomes more exaggerated as they squat or move onto one leg, this may be an area that deserves attention.

Conversely, if the individual has relatively well-aligned joint positions when standing, but optimal alignment is lost when you have them move, this may be an area you wish to evaluate further. Some of these individuals simply need to learn a more optimal movement strategy, whereas others may need physical intervention to help them develop a more optimal strategy. It is important to correlate postural findings with a movement assessment. Do not make assumptions or recommendations on the basis of posture alone.

2. When assessing movement it is often a challenge to decide where to focus one's attention, since there can be so many moving parts. Posture evaluation allows the clinician to:
   - assess for neutral alignment and joint centration;
   - identify the areas that seem most problematic (loss of neutral alignment, regions of non-optimal joint centration, regions of discomfort, areas of hyper- or hypotonicity) and focus on those regions as the individual begins to move;
   - establish a baseline posture for comparison purposes after a re-evaluation.

3. The position of the body in quiet standing is similar to that in the mid stance phase of gait. This is therefore a useful starting place when looking at the ability to ultimately support oneself in a single-leg stance and during gait.

There are, however, several challenges associated with using postural assessment as a valid evaluation tool:

1. *Using postural assessment as a stand-alone assessment.* The biggest fault with using postural assessment as a valid evaluation tool is that, too often, diagnoses/recommendations and subsequent treatment/corrective exercise programs are created solely on the basis of that assessment. As stated above, postural assessment should be just one element of a comprehensive evaluation. Postural assessment should always be followed up with a movement assessment, and should never be used in isolation to diagnose or develop a patient's or client's program.

2. *Casual observation and stereotyping of an individual's posture.* Ralph Waldo Emerson wrote: "People only see what they are prepared to see." This is such a true statement when it comes to evaluating posture. It is common for individuals (physicians, therapists, fitness professionals) to be trained in a certain evaluation and/or treatment method. The methods that have a greater tendency toward "cookbook" approaches usually lump everyone into a particular postural category. These approaches will often make claims such as "everyone has an anterior pelvic tilt, as everyone sits so much" or "everyone has an increased lumbar lordosis and thoracic kyphosis because of computers and smart phones." Therefore, upon casual observation the practitioner sees exactly what they have been trained to see.

It is important to recognize that the eyes only see what they have been trained to see. In other words, there is an education and clincal bias and; that information then "tricks" the eyes during postural evaluation. Additionally, because of biases and an individual's *anthropometrics* (their size and shape), the eyes are a very inaccurate tool in assessing posture. Palpation is a much more accurate evaluation, as they can actually feel where the bone(s) is/are located. One way to improve postural observation is to first take a general look at the individual; next, the clinician closes their eyes and palpates the region to get a sense of the position of the bones; then reopens their eyes and see if what they feel matches what they see. If placing one's hands on their client is outside the scope of practice then they will have to rely upon the eyes to detect postural issues. Just recognize that while one will likely be able to pick up some of the bigger issues, there may be some specific changes that are happening at the joint level that will be missed. In some situations, it can be helpful to refer the client to a practitioner who can perform a more skilled postural evaluation, identify and to address the underlying or true causes, rather than relying on superficial observations.

3. *Inter-tester reliability.* Each individual practitioner has a unique skill set in assessment, manual therapy, cuing, rehabilitation, and training. Likewise, depending on their training and experience, some practitioners are better at evaluating posture than others. Inter-tester reliability can therefore frequently be very poor, which is why postural assessment is often invalidated as a useful evaluation tool. Like most things, postural evaluation is a skill that can be honed after observing and palpating many different individuals. Unless a colleague is equally trained and skilled in assessment, the clinician should not allow others to invalidate their findings if they have followed a rational assessment process.

In order to make postural assessment a viable component of the assessment process, there are three keys to performing it thoroughly, accurately, and consistently:

1. The clinician should free their mind from preconceived notions. Developing an unbiased approach to postural assessment will enable one to better recognize what is there, rather than what one might think is there.

2. When evaluating posture, it is important that one evaluates the position of the bones and not where the overall body is located. One's perception, and therefore the accuracy of a visual assessment, can be altered by an individual's body size and shape—for example,

the presence/absence of muscle hypertrophy, the size of the breast tissue in females, the amount of adipose tissue, excessively large or small bone structure, the positions of their shoulders or head, their foot type (neutral, supinated, pronated, or a combination thereof), and their overall height. Even one's own body position and posture can affect what one sees. Therefore, the practitioner is encouraged to relax and square themselves to the individual they are assessing. After a cursory glance at their overall alignment, palpation is the most accurate way to determine a person's actual postural strategy.

3. Do not make assumptions or design a program strictly on the basis of the results of the postural evaluation. While important, posture is only one component of the client's or patient's overall evaluation. Combine the findings from the postural observations to see if it fits the findings from the other assessments, or to determine whether or not posture is a factor in the individual's overall movement strategy and their primary issues.

Neutral Alignment

Is there such a thing as 'optimal' or 'deal' posture? While research has attempted to determine normative values for posture, unfortunately it is challenging given varied history that each individual presents with as well as the set of parameters that different clinicians/therapists use to evaluate 'optimal' or 'ideal' posture. However, given these limitations it does not mean that postural evaluation should be completely discounted or that there is not an 'optimal' or 'ideal' strategy for posture. This concept is beautifully articulated in the book *Clinical Rehabilitation* (p. 37, Kolar et al. 2013):

"To define and 'ideal posture', we must, in our own approach, identify the biomechanical, anatomical, and neurophysiological functions and the interconnection of these functions in the context of motor or morphological development."

This book has defined 'optimal' posture based upon current understanding of anatomy, biomechanics, and motor control as well as child development. Additionally, it has been greatly influenced by studying with researchers and practitioners such as Dr. Linda-Joy Lee, Diane Lee, Dr. Paul Hodges, Shirley Sahrmann, Pavel Kolar, and the late Vladimir Janda.

The position of relative neutral joint alignment of the head, neck, TPC, and lower extremities that has been referenced throughout this book is described below. During postural evaluation it is best to have the individual stand against a blank wall, so that the background does not influence your vision. Have them march in place a few times and then assume a natural standing position, as this settles them into their typical posture.

Note: The landmarks described below are relative reference points rather than absolute exact positions.

- The head is supported upon the neck, and the neck is supported over the thorax.
  - A straight line running from the front of the orbit to the front of the mandible should be vertical to the floor.
- The thorax is supported and suspended over the pelvis.
  - The ribs should be aligned so that they are slightly higher at the back than at the front, and there should be spaces between the ribs.
- There is a slight lordotic cervical curve, kyphotic thoracic curve, and lordotic lumbar curve.
  - These curves should be present and gradual, without any exaggerated regions in either direction (too much or too little curvature).
- The pelvis is in a slight anterior pelvic tilt.
  - The anterior superior iliac spines (ASISs) are slightly forward of the pubic symphysis (this position may be altered in an individual who has spinal stenosis—they will tend to assume a more posterior pelvic tilt and have a flexed lumbar spine posture).

- The shoulders are open and wide through the front, and the scapulae rest flush on the thorax, with a slight upward rotation and posterior tilt.
  - The humeral head is just slightly forward of the front of the acromion process.
  - The arms hang straight and the palms should face the body when the individual is standing.
  - The elbow fossa face forward.
- The hips, knees, and ankles are aligned in a relatively straight line. It is important to use the following as relative points of reference:
  - From the side, a plumb line should fall slightly posterior to the greater trochanter, slightly anterior to the lateral knee, and slightly anterior to the lateral malleolus.
  - From the front, the straight line will be slightly angled from the hip, passing through the center of the patella and then through the second metatarsal of the foot.
  - From the rear, the line should be slightly angled from the hip, passing through

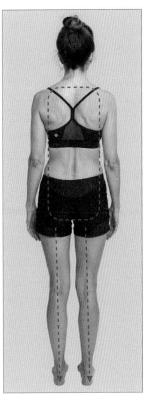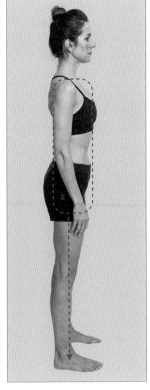

the center of the popliteal fossa, Achilles tendon, and then center of the calcaneus.

- The knees are aligned.
  - From the front, the patellae face straight forward.
  - From the rear, the popliteal fossae face straight backward.
- The feet are positioned hip-width apart, with the toes straight and the body weight supported primarily upon the five metatarsophalangeal joints and calcaneus.
  - The transverse, medial and longitudinal arches of the feet are maintained, with most of the body weight supported over the foot tripod: first metatarsophalangeal joint (big-toe side of the foot), fifth metatarsophalangeal joint (little-toe side of the foot), and calcaneus (heel).
  - The Achilles tendons are relatively vertical.

The postural assessment should be followed with a comprehensive evaluation appropriate to the practitioner's scope of practice (ranges of motion, muscle tests, tissue palpations, orthopedic/neurological tests, etc.).

Posture should be re-evaluated at the end of the corrective intervention to see if there are any noticeable changes. If the *primary driver,* the main issue causing the individual's non-optimal movement strategy, has been addressed, an improved postural alignment is often noted post-intervention. Of greater importance than whether or not the individual has better-looking posture is that they have an improved movement strategy to help them accomplish their functional goals with greater ease and efficiency. Generally, when the individual has developed a more optimal movement strategy, their postural strategy is also improved and they will appear more aligned.

Suspension

Concept of Suspension

The ability to stand, walk, and move requires a far more coordinated approach than simply contracting muscles to hold us in a fixed position or to perform a particular movement. When the neuromyofascial system is working as designed, the body is essentially suspended from the head, supported by internal pressure regulation, and strategically balanced from below upon the suspensory springs or arches of the feet. This ability to suspend is what enables the muscles to work as they should to coordinate stability and movement. Suspension enables one's body to move efficiently and relatively effortlessly, almost as if one were floating. A healthy young child playing in a carefree way, a well-trained dancer executing a dance performance, and an athlete performing a highly coordinated sporting activity and making it look easy all exemplify the use of suspension in creating efficient and relatively effortless movement.

Resistance training creates an additional compressive force upon the body. It is the ability to suspend that enables the body to essentially decompress itself under the forces of gravity, bodyweight, and external loads.

There are three components that ultimately contribute to achieving this degree of suspension:

1. *Proprioception and neuromuscular control.* The nervous system must coordinate activity throughout the body so the central nervous system receives/sends out the appropriate information from/to the myofascial system.
2. *The myofascial systems.* The fascial system essentially allows the body to be suspended and move without the exclusive need for muscle compression to remain stable. Fascia, invested in muscles, tendons, ligaments, and joint capsules, provides *tensegrity*, derived

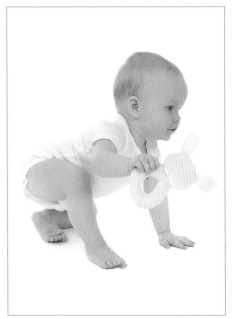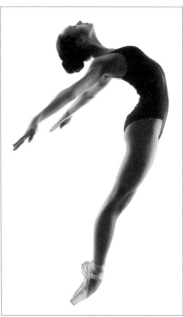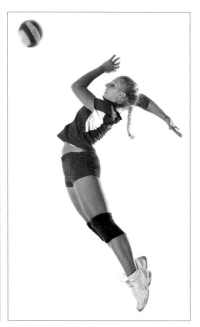

A healthy young child playing in a mobile, carefree manner, a well-trained dancer performing, and an athlete performing a highly coordinated sporting activity and making it look easy all exemplify the use of suspension in creating efficient and relatively effortless movement.

from the words tension and integrity, can be thought of as floating compression. In the tensegrity model of stability, bones are relatively floating and contained within the myofascial structures of the body. This inherent design of the body contributes significantly to the concept of suspension because the muscles fascially blending with other muscles and into ligaments, joint capsules, and bones and provides the body the ability to lengthen and retain stability.

Additionally, there must be an ability to seamlessly integrate the use of both the deep and the superficial myofascial systems, so that stabilization and movement demands are equally met using the most efficient strategy to complete the task. Neuromuscular control and balance between the deep and superficial myofascial systems enables the body to maintain relative alignment and joint centration throughout an infinite array of body movements and demands.

3. *Three-dimensional breathing.* Three-dimensional breathing is the body's inherent strategy for decompression. Three-dimensional breathing regulates pressure within the thoracic, abdominal, and pelvic cavities, and serves to provide internal support against external loads and contraction of the muscles that surround these regions. Without an optimal three-dimensional breathing strategy, the trunk, spine, and/or pelvis will become over-compressed and compensations will occur.

Role of the Psoas in Achieving Suspension

The psoas plays a critical role in the ability to achieve suspension of the trunk and spine. As discussed throughout this book, the psoas stabilizes the thoracolumbar junction and lumbar spine. The psoas anchors the spinal attachments of the diaphragm and pelvic floor, thereby supporting the muscles of respiration in breathing and pressure regulation through the thoracic, abdominal, and pelvic cavities.

Recognizing Signs of Non-optimal Suspension

A common reason for the inability to suspend is myofascial gripping. Gripping or chronic overactivity of the rectus abdominis and/or oblique abdominals leads to trunk and spinal flexion. Similarly, gripping or chronic overactivity of the latissimus dorsi and/or superficial erector spinae often causes over-compression of the posterior aspect of the trunk and spine. Both abdominal gripping and back gripping limit three-dimensional breathing and will ultimately over-compress the trunk, spine, and pelvis.

There are three additional common signs that indicate a non-optimal suspension strategy:

1. *Altered breathing strategy and chronic rib cage rigidity, low back, and/or hip tightness.* Clients who complain of chronic tightness, stiffness, and/or rigidity in their trunk, spine, and/or hips frequently have a poor ability to suspend or decompress their body. They will frequently have gripping around the trunk, spine, pelvis, and/or hip regions; quite often they will also demonstrate altered breathing techniques because of poor, or a lack of an efficient three-dimensional breathing strategy.

2. *Very restricted and "muscled"-type movements.* Many individuals use far too much muscular effort to perform very simple tasks, such as sitting or standing. This is generally why individuals complain about experiencing stiffness, discomfort, and/or fatigue after prolonged sitting or standing—they actually sit or stand in a posture that demands too much effort.

   Additionally, many individuals use excessive muscular activity during relatively simple movements, such as walking, body weight squatting, and similar exercises. This overuse is often related to the previously mentioned habitual compensations secondary to trauma,

injuries, and surgery. However, muscle overactivity can also be related to actively trying to "feel" muscles working during exercises, thus encouraging the individual to use more effort than is necessary to perform the pattern. Over time, this muscle overactivity becomes part of the individual's postural and movement habits.

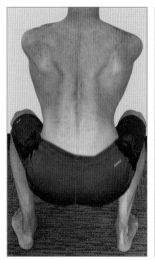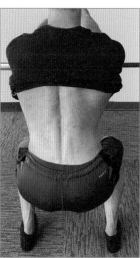

This individual presented with low back and hip pain affecting his ability to squat and deadlift. Note the difference in the erector tone while doing a body weight squat (left image) versus the supported version of the body weight squat (right image). While the erectors are required to support the trunk and pelvis during a squatting pattern, the strategy this individual is initially using requires far too much muscular demands than is required to perform the activity. The supported variation of the pattern allows him to focus on alignment, breathing, and control (suspension) while reducing the need for so much muscular activity. He will then work on replicating this reduced muscular activity as he performs the pattern without support.

3. *Abdominal distension and increased resting tone in the lower abdomen.* When the individual is unable to suspend, there will often be a

downwardly directed force during exertion. This is a type of Valsalva maneuver (a bearing down) when the individual is exerting force, such as when lifting a child, sitting up from a supine position, or performing an exercise. With this non-optimal strategy, the thoracic and abdominal organs will tend to displace inferiorly and create a distended appearance of the lower abdominal region. This appearance is often blamed on "weak" lower abdominals; however, on palpation the lower abdominal region is usually highly toned, because it is maintained in a habitually over-lengthened state. This strategy can often contribute to abdominal muscle strains and tears, groin 'pulls' and *diastasis recti*, or a longitudinal separation of the rectus abdominis.

Lower abdominal distension and abdominal oblique over-activity (arrow) in a patient with chronic left abdominal, groin, and hip pain (left and middle images below); hernia and other abdominal/pelvic organ pathology was ruled out in this individual with diastasis recti (right image below). These are common clinical signs, especially in active individuals, of an ineffective suspension strategy created by non-optimal internal pressure regulation and overuse of the superficial muscles for trunk and spine (core) stability.

Achieving Suspension

For many individuals experiencing chronic tension, rigidity, and discomfort, the most important strategy for changing these chronic habits is to teach them a more optimal suspension strategy. Many of the strategies to achieve suspension featured throughout this book can be summarized as follows:

- Think about suspension in the upright position in terms of imagining being gently lifted toward the ceiling by wires attached to the back of the head and ribs. There should be an overall feeling or sensation of lightness through the trunk and spine when holding the body in this manner.
- Utilize verbal and visualization cues, such as "Elongate or lengthen from the back of the spine, while keeping the front of the rib cage soft." Avoid cues like "Brace," "Squeeze," "Tighten," or "Tuck," as these tend to create more compression through the TPC.
- Encourage the client to perform a self-assessment, or "check in" with their body, and relax the areas where they are experiencing tension. Have them check in with the following regions, which are common areas of gripping that were not discussed earlier in this book:
  - Soften and relax their abdominals to release abdominal tension.

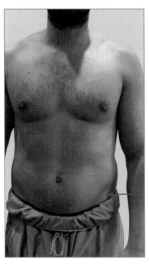 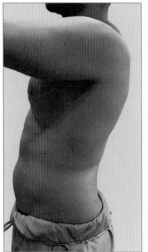

Lower abdominal distension.

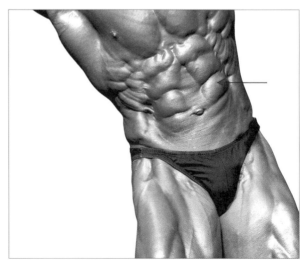

Diastasis recti.

- Relax and create space under their arms to reduce latissimus dorsi gripping, which is a common cause of neck, shoulder, and upper back tension.
  - Relax their toes and spread their feet to release chronic foot gripping.
- Maintain the visual cue that works best for the individual; they should then take a few three-dimensional breaths, imagining a ball or balloon being inflated inside their TPC. Breathing this way will expand the thorax and pelvic cavities and elongate the spine, without creating a change in neutral alignment.
- The individual continues with visualizations of being suspended and breathing three-dimensionally for 3–5 breath cycles. They should repeat this frequently throughout the day to encourage suspension and reduce chronic gripping. This is also an effective strategy for encouraging suspension during a workout, either prior to or after exercising.

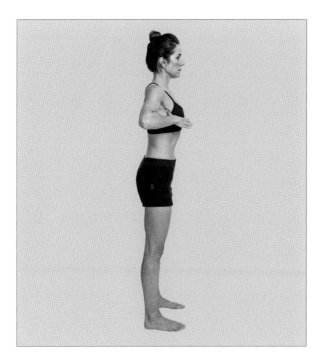

An effective strategy for promoting suspension is to have the individual place their thumbs in their axilla (armpits) and focus their breath into that region (image above). They will visualize being long through their spine and breathing into their

TPC and then maintain the sensation of being suspended as they are sitting, standing, and/or exercising.

For demonstration of how to create suspension, visit www.IIHFE.com/the-psoas-solution.

Be sure to integrate these concepts into a variety of positions and tasks. Naturally, during an externally loaded activity, such as a squat or deadlift pattern, the ability to remain suspended will be less than when the body is not loaded. However, the ultimate goal of achieving this sensation of suspension is to not allow the trunk and spine to be over-compressed during the exercise being performed.

Individuals who have a very compressed system can also benefit from a combination of myofascial release (either self-myofascial release and/or manual therapy work), breath training, postural education that encourages elongation and maintaining their alignment with less overall effort, and exercise cuing that encourages less compression, exertion, or forcefulness in their exercise. While it often takes time to change chronic habits, the use of a specific and consistent approach generally results in positive results.

The Pelvic Floor and Its Relationship to the Psoas

The pelvic floor is an important myofascial structure in the stabilization of the thoracopelvic cylinder (TPC) as well in bowel, bladder, and sexual functions. Until recently not much attention had been paid to the pelvic floor, and millions of individuals suffered in silence with incontinence and sexual dysfunction, and with stabilization issues of the TPC and hips. The pelvic floor has now garnered the much-needed attention it deserves, and there has been an advent of pelvic floor specialists to address these pelvis-related issues. While it is beyond the scope of this book to discuss this topic in depth, it is worth noting how the pelvic floor functions in conjunction with the psoas in stabilization and posture.

Functional Anatomy of the Pelvic Floor

The pelvic floor is arranged in three layers: (1) the endopelvic fascia, (2) the pelvic diaphragm, and (3) the urogenital diaphragm (Carrière 2002):

- The first layer, or *endopelvic fascia*, comprises smooth muscle, fascia, and ligaments that support the pelvic organs.
- The second layer is referred to as the *pelvic diaphragm*. The primary muscle of this layer, the levator ani, is considered by Carrière to be the most important in this region. The other muscles within this layer are: pubococcygeus, puborectalis, pubovaginalis (in females), levator prostatae (in males), iliococcygeus, coccygeus, and internal sphincter muscles of the bladder and rectum. This layer contains approximately 70% slow-twitch fibers and 30% fast-twitch fibers; it is primarily responsible for continence (control of urine and feces) and for supporting the anus, vagina, and prostate and the stability of the sacroiliac joint.
- The third layer, referred to as the *urogenital diaphragm*, consists of several muscles: deep transverse perineal, superficial transverse perineal, bulbospongiosus, ischiocavernosus, and anal sphincter. These muscles support the levator ani, continence, and sexual function.

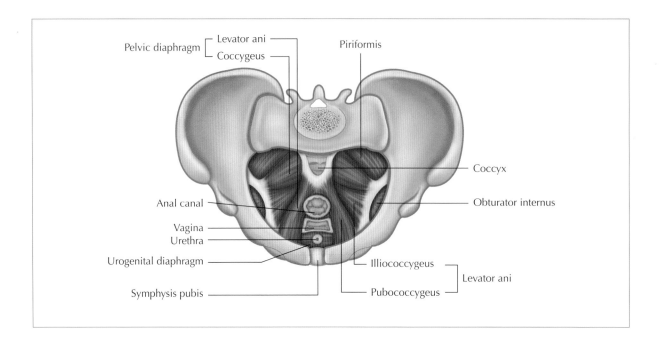

Role of the Pelvic Floor

There are three primary functions of the pelvic floor muscles:

1. *Pelvic organ support.* The pelvic floor supports the pelvic organs. The muscles of the pelvic floor must be strong enough to eccentrically contract to control the descent of the pelvic organs during inhalation, and then lift the organs back up during exhalation. When lifting, coughing, sneezing, and/or laughing, these muscles must quickly contract to maintain bowel and bladder continence.
2. *Sphincter control.* The pelvic floor muscles control the bladder and anal sphincters to ensure continence; when relaxed they allow urination and defecation. These muscles also support healthy function of the sexual organs.
3. *Pelvic and hip stabilization.* The pelvic floor muscles work with the respiratory diaphragm, psoas, and abdominal muscles to regulate internal pressure, which helps stabilize the pelvis and hips. In the breathing chapter (Chapter 2) it was discussed how the diaphragm and pelvic floor work in tandem— they lower during inspiration and rise during expiration. Additionally, in individuals with no evidence of pelvic floor muscle dysfunction, the pelvic floor and transversus abdominis co-activate to stabilize the lumbopelvic-hip complex (Sapsford et al. 2001).

As discussed in the functional anatomy chapter (Chapter 1), the psoas fascially blends into the pelvic floor. While there has been no research carried out to evaluate the combined roles of the psoas and pelvic floor, it is hypothesized that the psoas helps stabilize the lumbar spine and pelvis, so that contraction of the diaphragm and pelvic floor are coordinated and efficient (Osar 2015).

Signs of Non-optimal Use of the Pelvic Floor

There are three primary signs that indicate non-optimal function of the pelvic floor:

1. *Urinary incontinence.* Leakage of urine is the most common sign of pelvic floor dysfunction. It is often thought that incontinence is an issue that affects women only after childbirth and as they age. However, studies have

shown incontinence to be common in elite nulliparous (never having given birth) female athletes, with a reported rate of occurrence of 28–45% (Poswiata et al. 2014, Thyssen et al. 2002, Nygaard et al. 1994). Pelvic floor training has been shown to improve pelvic floor function and continence in most populations that have been prescribed specific exercises to target these particular muscles.

2. *Hip gripping and posterior pelvic tilt.* As discussed in Appendix VI (Sitting), a slumped posture—posterior pelvic tilt and lumbar spine flexion—is extremely common in many people when sitting. Posterior hip gripping (superficial gluteus maximus, hip rotators, and/or hamstrings) and superficial abdominal gripping (external/internal obliques and rectus abdominis) respectively pull the pelvis into a posterior pelvic tilt and flex the lumbar spine. Either of these conditions makes it impossible to assume an upright sitting posture without compensating by overextending in the thoracic spine. This undesirable sitting strategy perpetuates muscle imbalances, including inhibition of the psoas and pelvic floor, which subsequently lead to non-optimal TPC stabilization and breathing dysfunction. Interestingly, individuals standing in a hypolordotic posture (generally associated with a posterior pelvic tilt) demonstrated a higher resting tone of the pelvic floor, suggesting overactivity of these muscles, than when standing in either a neutral or hyperlordotic posture (Capson et al. 2011). Retraining control of neutral alignment in a variety of positions can improve the function of not only the pelvic floor but also the psoas. As reported by Sapsford et al. (2008), both continent and incontinent women who sat more upright (i.e. assumed a position approximating neutral lumbar spine and pelvic alignment) tended to have greater pelvic floor activation than those who sat in a slumped posture. In this book several strategies have been discussed for improving alignment and control of the lumbar spine, pelvis, and hips, as well as for restoring function of the deep myofascial system (DMS) (e.g. psoas, transversus abdominis, and pelvic floor).

3. *Pelvic pain syndrome.* Pelvic pain syndrome (PPS) includes pain that originates from the joints, myofascia, or organs within the pelvis. PPS affects the ability to optimally recruit the pelvic floor, and can also impact breathing and activation of the DMS. Most individuals experiencing PPS require the services of a pelvic floor specialist to address the pain component as well as identify the cause. Specific retraining of the pelvic floor muscles (the entire DMS), restoring three-dimensional breathing, and incorporating the corresponding strategies into the activities of daily living and exercise can help those individuals improve function and reduce symptoms.

Improving activation of the pelvic floor as part of an overall core stabilization strategy was discussed in the breathing chapter (Chapter 2). For more detailed information on this topic, readers are encouraged to consult the works of Lee (2012), Hodges et al. (2013), Richardson et al. (2004), Sapsford et al. (2008, 2001), and Carrière (2002).

Psoas' Role in Femoroacetabular Impingement (FAI) and Labral Pathologies of the Hip

Topics

- Femoroacetabular impingement and labral pathologies of the hip
- Psoas' role in hip centration
- Identifying signs of non-optimal use of the psoas and centration of the hip

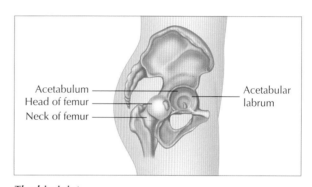

The hip joint.

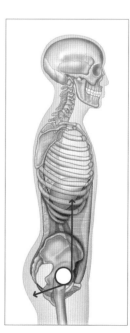

The psoas draws the femoral head superiorly and deep, lower fibers of gluteus maximus draw the femoral head posteriorly to help control of the femoral head within the acetabulum.

Many individuals presenting with reduced range of motion in the hip, loss of strength, pain, and/or degraded performance have an internal hip derangement. Two common causes of these issues are labral tears and femoroacetabular impingement (FAI). This section will briefly discuss the psoas' involvement in these two issues.

The hip joint is formed by the femoral head of the femur articulating with the acetabulum, or the socket. The labrum of the hip is a fibrocartilaginous structure that surrounds the acetabulum, deepening the socket; it creates almost a suction-cup effect around the femoral head, an effect which likely plays a role in stabilizing the joint (Osar 2015). When there is balance between the deep and superficial

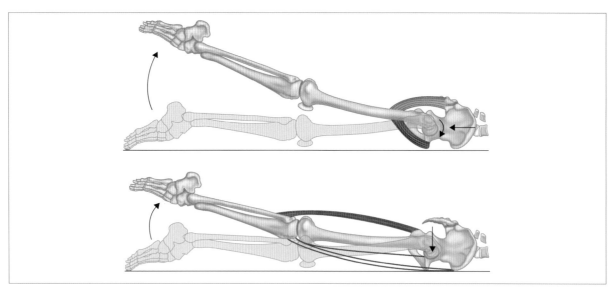

Optimal co-activation of the deep and superficial myofascial system provide centration so extension occurs directly around the hip joint itself allowing the femoral head to rotate within the acetabulum (top image). With inhibition of the psoas, gluteus, or other deep muscles of the hip, the hamstrings assume the primary role of hip extension and subsequently drive the femoral head forward during hip extension (bottom image). This is a common presentation in individuals with chronic hamstring issues, labral tears and FAI.

myofascial systems, the femoral head remains centrated within the acetabulum; this ensures optimal strength and range of motion, and decreases the risk of soft tissue injury.

A common cause of hip problems—in particular, anterior pinching and discomfort with hip flexion, adduction, and/or internal rotation—is an impingement of soft tissue and/or bony structures within the joint. Although soft tissues, such as the labrum, psoas tendon, and joint capsule, can be pinched, FAI technically occurs when there is bony impingement between the femoral head and the acetabulum.

There are three types of FAI: pincer, cam, and a combination thereof.

- A *pincer lesion* is where an overgrowth of the acetabulum covers the femoral head and "pinches" it during certain hip movements (image left).
- A *cam lesion* is where an overgrowth around the femoral head and/or neck creates impingement during certain hip movements (image middle).
- A *combination* of the pincer and cam lesions occurs when an overgrowth is present on both the acetabulum and the femoral head/neck (image right).

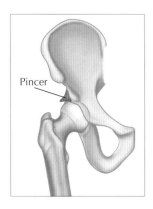
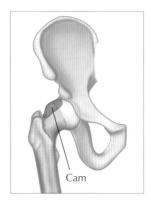
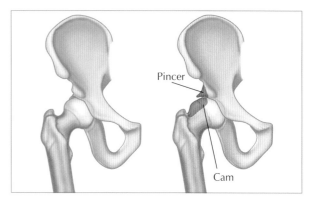

Additionally, bony growths can impinge on the psoas tendon, joint capsule, and/or labrum, and lead to significant discomfort and inefficient performance. Patients will generally complain of deep, non-specific hip pain or pinching sensations in certain ranges of motion; they may also have a habit of cupping their hand in the shape of the letter C (known as the "C sign") around the outside of their pelvis and thigh. The pain generally worsens with prolonged sitting and tends to be progressive in nature. Conventional treatment for FAI is anti-inflammatory medication, rest, physical therapy, and/or arthroscopic surgery (Kuhlman and Domb 2009, Dooley 2008).

Another common cause of hip dysfunction and pain is soft tissue impingement and labral tears (see image below). These impingement syndromes and tears of the acetabular labrum are often blamed on the psoas (Blankenbaker et al. 2012, Hwang et al. 2015, Nelson and Keene 2014, Dobbs et al. 2002, Taylor and Clarke 1995). As a result, arthroscopic release of the iliopsoas tendon is becoming an increasingly recommended treatment for acetabular impingement, as well as for "snapping" hip syndrome, a condition where the psoas tendon "snaps" within the pelvis or groin region (Hwang et al. 2015, Nelson and Keene 2014, Dobbs et al. 2002, Taylor and Clarke 1995).

Unfortunately, there have been no follow-up studies to indicate the long-term effects of these types of surgery on hip and/or spine function

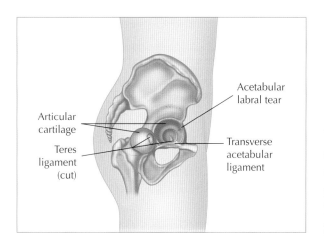

Articular cartilage

Teres ligament (cut)

Acetabular labral tear

Transverse acetabular ligament

(most studies cover a two- or three-year post-surgical period, and there are few, if any, studies relating to periods of more than five years after surgery). However, in a follow-up investigation of individuals who underwent arthroscopic iliopsoas release within the previous three years, both atrophy (25% decrease in size) and decreased muscle strength in hip flexion were noted (Brandenburg et al. 2016).

There are several potential risks associated with these invasive types of procedure:

1. The underlying factor driving the initial problem is likely not an isolated psoas issue; releasing the psoas tendon does not therefore change the driving factor of the issue. Just as the psoas is never the only muscle involved in proper hip function, it is rarely (if ever) the sole muscle responsible for a dysfunction.

2. In many individuals, non-optimal hip centration and TPC alignment contribute to their hip issues. Not only will releasing the psoas tendon fail to solve these individuals' issues, but it will also make it virtually impossible for them to develop optimal hip function. The strategies described in this book have been used to successfully treat countless numbers of patients who have been diagnosed with psoas issues, labral tears, and snapping hips.

3. While more research and long-term follow up is required, there is evidence that surgery and related interventions may contribute to advancing degenerative changes (Salata et al. 2010, Gruber et al. 2012). Naturally, there are obvious situations where addressing the current problem (pain, weakness, dysfunction) outweigh the potential long-term risks of surgery.

There are indeed individuals who certainly require surgery to resolve their issues; however, many of them are given a surgical recommendation before the underlying causes of their problems have been properly identified. As with any surgical intervention, it is important the individual gets several opinions and follows an appropriate course of conservative treatment prior to surgical procedure. Once a muscle is cut (released), it cannot be reattached, and that whatever function that muscle was responsible for, its role will be diminished, which will necessitate compensation by other muscles.

Assessing for Impingement

The Impingement, or FADIR (flexion, adduction, internal rotation), test is helpful for detecting if there is impingement of the psoas tendon, joint capsule, and/or labrum, or if FAI is present.

Procedure

- The individual lies supine, with their arms and legs straight.
- The tester flexes the individual's hip and knee to approximately 90° (flexible individuals can be flexed to more than 90°), adducts their femur across the midline, and internally rotates their hip (image below).

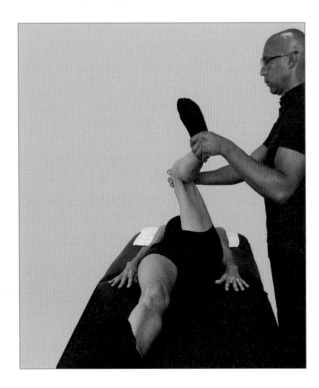

- A positive test is the occurrence of pain or a "pinching" sensation in the anterior hip or groin region.

The impingement test does not differentiate between issues of the hip related to soft tissue and those related to bony structures. Research suggests that there are positive signs of FAI present in up to 95% of individuals experiencing a labral tear (Yazbek et al. 2011); moreover, the anterior, superior region of the hip joint has been found to be the most common location of these tears (Yazbek et al. 2011). Interestingly, significant posterior and/or lateral hip gripping will cause the femoral head to translate anteriorly and superiorly. Clinically, many patients being evaluated with hip pain, who demonstrated a positive impingement test, and suspected labral tear, have presented with an anteriorly and superiorly positioned femoral head. Most of these individuals tested positive in the impingement test, even in situations were there was no sign of FAI on radiographs or MRIs.

Many of individuals can be treated conservatively and do not require surgery. There are three keys to developing a more optimal hip strategy, improving function, and decreasing pain in these individuals:

1. *Stop gripping.* In many individuals with hip problems, it is usually more important to stop the non-optimal habits than to develop greater strength and flexibility. As mentioned, many individuals experiencing labral tears and hip impingement are over-gripping (chronically over-contracting) their posterior hip muscles (superficial gluteus maximus, hip rotators, posterior fibers of gluteus medius, hamstrings) and are driving their femoral head forward and/or superiorly. This strategy inhibits the psoas and deeper fibers of the gluteus maximus, thereby disrupting optimal hip centration.

   Myofascial gripping is often an unconscious process that has developed secondarily to reflexive compensations or consciously trained habits (too much focus on "squeezing," or overtightening, muscles during the concentric phase of an exercise pattern). Gripping can also be a postural strategy for holding oneself in better postural alignment and/or for making one's stomach or glutes appear smaller—in other words, it is an attempt to make an area of the body look more aesthetically appealing.

Without a conscious awareness to stop a gripping pattern, no amount of stretching or strengthening exercise will provide long-term improvements in an individual's presentation or symptoms. These individuals must be made aware that they are gripping, and then taught how to consciously relax the muscles in question throughout the day.

The self-assessment procedure for determining whether or not one is hip gripping and the self-release is as follows:

- The individual stands and places their hands on either side of their pelvis, cupping the glutes and hip muscles to get a sense of the amount of tone in those muscles: at rest, they should be soft and relaxed.
- They will then slide their hands down the outside of your hips. A relaxed and well-developed gluteal muscle should be round and full, not contracted and hollow. If they notice hollowing in the lateral or posterior gluteal region, they are likely a hip gripper (and over-contracting their hips).
- To release chronic gripping, the individual takes a deep breath in and contracts their glutes. They, release the breath and visualize spreading their ischial tuberosities (sits bones).
- Reassess the hips—they should now feel more relaxed and soft; that is how they should feel throughout the day in quiet standing and sitting, and when not being actively used.
- To stop chronic hip gripping, this relaxation technique must become a conscious habit and be practiced consistently until the hips are more relaxed while at rest. Body weight squatting while focusing on breathing and relaxation of the hips—focus on softening the front of the hips and widening through the back of the hips—is an effective strategy for maintaining relaxed hips (image below right).

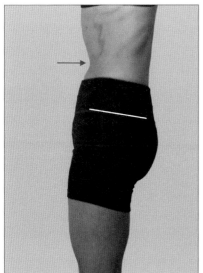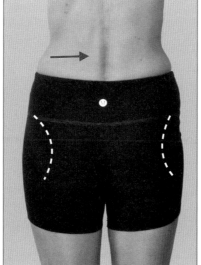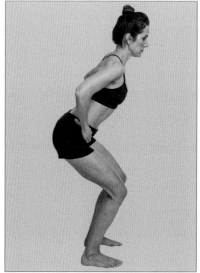

Abdominal gripping (left); Hip gripping (middle); both strategies tend to posteriorly rotate the pelvis, flex the lumbar spine, and drive the femoral head anteriorly. Chronically maintaining this strategy is a common contributor to soft tissue impingement of the hip and FAI.

See video on Squatting: www.IIHFE.com/the-psoas-solution

2. *Apply the foundational ABCs.* The use of the foundational ABCs—alignment, breathing, and control—was discussed in this book in the development and restoration of ideal psoas function and hip centration. Optimal hip centration must be incorporated into exercise, as well as into daily habits, in order to ensure that the individual is able to successfully adopt and maintain more optimal postural and movement strategies.

3. *Train appropriately.* Many individuals experiencing chronic hip issues are exercising too frequently and/or too intensely; they might also be performing exercises at a level too high for their current level of ability to control their trunk, spine, pelvis, and/or hips. Additionally, many of these same individuals are performing progressive exercise without paying enough attention to their ABCs, as well as using inappropriate cuing to activate their glutes, abdominals, and other core/hip muscles. As noted above, this will inhibit the psoas and affect hip centration.

Have the individual focus on maintaining their ABCs, and use the most appropriate movement patterns and progressions. Ensure that individuals are progressed safely by using a suitable frequency and intensity, along with proper cuing. Maintaining optimal ABCs throughout a corrective and functional exercise program, while using the most appropriate exercise patterns and cuing, will then will give your patients and clients the best opportunity for achieving a successful outcome.

Sitting

Because so many people all over the world now work on computers or smart devices, a discussion of the topic of sitting is warranted. Although most individuals would benefit from using a standing desk, or from at least interspersing periods of time sitting with periods of standing, the reality is that nearly everyone who participates in modern culture will spend a great deal of their life in a seated position.

While there are many health disadvantages associated with the seated position, many of the musculoskeletal problems have more to do with the individual's posture when seated than with the act of sitting itself. This section will discuss the role of the psoas in sitting, as well as a strategy for developing a more optimal sitting strategy; some common signs of a non-optimal sitting strategy will be highlighted.

Psoas' Role in Sitting

There are three primary roles of the psoas in sitting:

1. The psoas stabilizes the thoracolumbar junction (TLJ) and lumbar spine; this helps maintain optimal alignment of the trunk and spine over the pelvis.
2. The psoas helps maintain a neutral alignment of the pelvis (anterior pelvic tilt), which helps align and support the spine above it.
3. By virtue of its fascial connections to the diaphragm and pelvic floor, the psoas supports an optimal three-dimensional breathing strategy while in the seated position, allowing the individual to regulate internal pressures and maintain suspension.

Teaching an Optimal Sitting Strategy

Three keys to developing an optimal sitting strategy are presented below. This strategy works best when sitting in an office chair, because the height can be adjusted; however, it should also be used when sitting in a car, on a couch, or in a restaurant.

1. *Align the thoracopelvic cylinder (TPC).*
   - While standing, the individual aligns and stacks their thorax over their pelvis. They visualize a wire gently pulling them from the back of their head toward the ceiling. They should be visualizing an elongation of their spine and creating space in between their ribs, without lifting the chest up. For more information about this postural position, see Appendix III (Suspension).

2. *Hinge at the hips.*
   - While maintaining neutral alignment of their TPC, the individual hinges or flexes at the hips.
   - They continue to flex the hips, knees, and ankles, sending their pelvis back until they are seated; essentially, they are squatting onto the chair. A good cue is to have them think about "releasing through their posterior hip" or "spreading their sits bones." For more information about this postural position and relevant cuing refer back to the chapter about squatting (Chapter 4).
   - They should end up perched upon their pelvis, which helps maintain a neutral pelvis position, instead of trying to sit their back all the way against the back of the chair. They should effectively be resting upon their "sits bones" (ischial tuberosities), rather than upon their sacrum. Only allow them to position themselves against the back of the chair if they are able to maintain this alignment. Individuals with shorter legs may need a foot support to help align themselves in this position.

3. *Spread the sits bones (ischial tuberosities).*
   - This technique (which is a modified version learned from Diane Lee, PT and Dr. Linda-Joy Lee, Ph.D., PT) is incredibly effective in assisting the individual with better positioning their pelvis and hips. Once seated, the individual cups their hands under their upper thigh and gently pulls up, out, and back, and then repeats on the other leg. This is an extremely effective strategy for aligning and positioning the pelvis in a more neutral or anteriorly tilted position, while centrating the hip. For a demonstration of the technique,

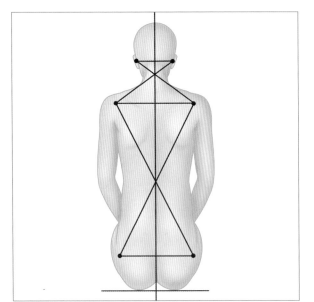 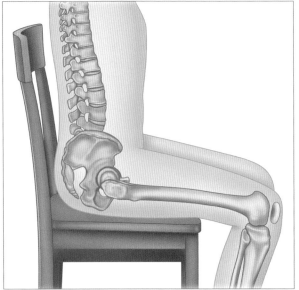

The head and spine supported upon the ischial tuberosities (sits bones) helps to promote postural efficiency. Neutral pelvic alignment supports optimal lordotic curvature of the lumbar spine (right image).

visit the website www.IIHFE.com/
the-psoas-solution.

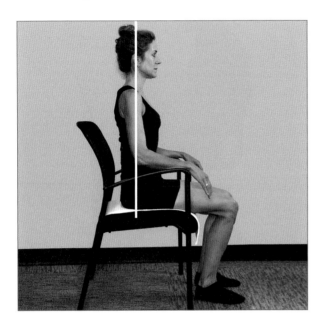

An optimal sitting strategy supports the trunk on top of the pelvis and promotes neutral spinal alignment. Note the general alignment of the head and truck over the pelvis as well as the relative lordotic position of the spine in the image above. The individual's bodyweight is supported primarily upon her ischial tuberosities (sits bones).

Signs of a Non-optimal Sitting Strategy

There are three common signs of a non-optimal sitting strategy:

1. The thorax is positioned behind the pelvis.
2. The pelvis is positioned in a posterior pelvic tilt.
3. The lumbar spine is in flexion, with either excessive flexion at the thoracolumbar junction (TLJ) or an increased thoracic lordosis.

Several factors can lead to this non-optimal sitting posture:

1. Most chairs are designed to position the thorax behind the pelvis as the back of the chair is positioned behind the seat. Also, many chairs and most couches are designed where the knees are positioned higher than the hips so there is a greater likelihood of posterior pelvic tilt and lumbar spine flexion.
2. Many individuals have poor hip mobility and are positioned in a posterior pelvic tilt. As a result of this, combined with a general lack of awareness of where neutral alignment is, they sit with a persistent posterior pelvic tilt for the majority of their lives. The posterior pelvic tilt then pulls the lumbar spine into flexion,

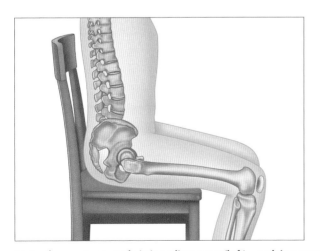
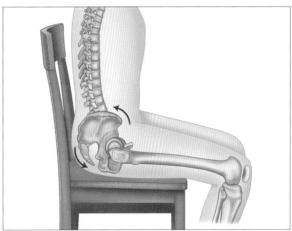

Note the more neutral sitting alignment (left)—pelvis neutral and lumbar lordosis and the weight is primarily upon the ischial tuberosities of the pelvis—and the typical sitting posture above right characterized by posterior rotation of the pelvis and lumbar spine flexion with the weight behind the ischial tuberosities (right).

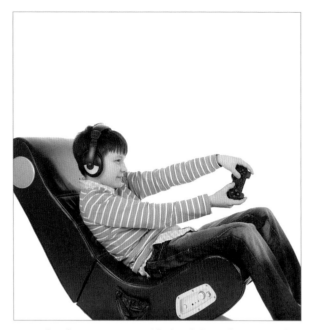 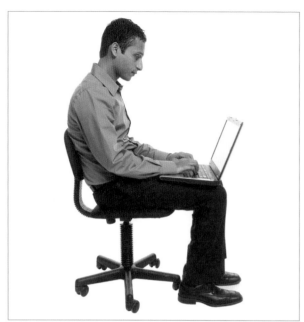

Note the thorax positioned behind the pelvis, spinal flexion, and posterior pelvic tilt position in two examples of common seated postures when playing video games (left) and working on a laptop computer (right).

thereby decreasing the natural lordotic curve of the lumbar spine.

3. To accommodate these changes and to remain upright, the individual will often extend excessively, either at the TLJ or through the upper thorax.

The non-optimal sitting posture will contribute to (and perpetuate) the following changes in the TPC and the hips:

- Shortness and tightness in the superficial fibers of the gluteus maximus, hamstrings, rectus abdominis, and oblique abdominals, which keeps the individual in a posterior pelvic tilt and lumbar spine flexion.
- Shortness and tightness in the thoracolumbar and/or upper thoracic erector spinae, thereby perpetuating extension and rigidity in these regions.
- Inability to achieve optimal three-dimensional breathing, since the thorax is not properly stacked over the pelvis, and the excessive thoracolumbar and/or thoracic extension inhibits proper use of the posterior aspect of the diaphragm.

- Inhibition of the psoas and deep myofascial system, because of non-optimal TPC alignment and altered breathing habits, leading to non-optimal positional control of the lumbar spine, pelvis, and hips.
- Overstretched hip flexors[1], which, in combination with the short hamstrings and superficial glutes, perpetuates posterior pelvic tilt and lumbar spine flexion.

Over time, this postural position overloads the intervertebral discs, overstretches the posterior ligaments and joint capsules of the lumbar spine and sacroiliac joints, and overstretches neural structures (dura and nerve roots of the lumbar spine). These gradually lead to lumbar and pelvic pain, discogenic pathology (bulges and herniations), sciatica (irritation of the sciatic nerve), and neuralgia (nerve pain); they also

---

[1]Overstretched muscles are often overactive (hypertonic), as they are attempting to counteract their functional antagonists; in this case, the hip flexors are counteracting the pull of the superficial glutes and hamstrings. This causes the individual to experience the sensation of their hip flexors being overly "tight." They are overstretched and "feel" tight, rather than actually being too short.

perpetuate a host of muscle imbalances around the trunk, pelvis, and lower extremities.

While not always easy to perform because of chair design, the best way to self-correct a non-optimal sitting strategy is as follows:

- Stand up and reposition the TPC as described above. Maintain the sensation of being suspended from the back of the head as well as from the posterior aspect of the spine and thorax.
- Take 5 three-dimensional breaths, focusing on breathing into the back of the rib cage.
- Perform 5 repetitions of the Supported Squat pattern using the edge of a desk or table for support. Focus on releasing and sitting back into the hips.
- Reposition oneself on the chair using the squat strategy described above.
- Take frequent mini-breaks to reposition the body and to minimize the risks associated with a long-term seated position. For the majority of individuals who sit for the best part of the day, this is often the most important of all the aforementioned strategies.

For a video demonstration of how to develop an optimal sitting strategy, visit the website www.IIHFE.com/the-psoas-solution.

Corrective Exercise

"Corrective exercise" is a term that has come into vogue in the last decade. Depending on whom one speaks with, one is bound to get many different opinions about what it is and how to implement it into training programs. Like its predecessors *core training* and *functional training*, corrective exercise has been poorly defined. It is most often associated with self-myofascial release techniques (such as foam rolling, stretching, or mobility work), and rehabilitation-influenced exercises (such as breathing, Bird-Dogs, and Bridges). While corrective exercise may include these modalities,

the approach presented in this book—the Integrative Movement System Corrective Exercise Strategy™—entails a very specific method for integrating corrective exercise into clients' and patients' programs.

Why is there even a need for corrective exercise? It really boils down to one key reason: habits. What is a habit? A habit is: "a behavior or pattern acquired by frequent repetition or physiological exposure that shows itself in regularity or increased facility of performance" (source: http://www.merriam-webster.com/dictionary/habit).

An individual's postural and movement habits have become ingrained by a variety of factors, including:

- Things taught by parents, teachers, health practitioners, and/or coaches.
- Conscious or unconscious compensations developed following injury, trauma, or surgery.
- Things learned from observations of parents, teachers, coaches, etc., especially early in development.
- The types of exercises performed.
- Prolonged physical inactivity.

- Occupation and the repetitive patterns developed as a result.
- Emotions—more confident individuals generally assume a very different posture than individuals who are chronically depressed or have been the victim of physical, sexual, or verbal abuse.
- Pain—especially if chronic in nature, will always affect one's posture and movement strategy.
- Low energy levels and fatigue—these can often make it challenging to utilize muscles appropriately for posture and movement.

One of the most important responsibilities as health and fitness professionals is to help patients/clients identify their current non-optimal habits that are contributing to their current dysfunction and/or inefficient performance. From this information then help them develop more optimal habits and move them toward achieving their health and fitness goals.

The Integrative Movement System Corrective Exercise Strategy™

As the name suggests, the Integrative Movement System Corrective Exercise Strategy™ is an approach (rather than a series of exercises) aimed at identifying the key factors contributing to an individual's current non-optimal posture and movement habits. It incorporates assessment and subsequently the thoughtful implementation of specific release and/or activation techniques to address an individual's primary issue(s) that is/are driving their chronic problems or degraded performance (these are the factors that are directly contributing to postural and movement dysfunction, loss of strength, and/or decreased performance). The specific corrective exercises utilized in this book incorporate the principles of the Integrative Movement System™—namely, alignment, breathing, and control—to improve an individual's postural and movement habits.

In this approach, corrective exercise is not meant to fix or correct an individual's posture or movement. Nor is it designed to replace a fundamentally sound training or conditioning program. An equally important part of the Integrative Movement System Corrective Exercise Strategy™ is not only to identify and address the factors that are contributing to an individual's non-optimal posture and/or movement habits, but also to incorporate these changes into the fundamental movement patterns—squatting, lunging, bending, rotating, pushing, pulling, balance, and gait—so that the individual can efficiently accomplish their health and fitness goals. Corrective exercise is therefore not intended as a replacement of a well-designed strength and conditioning program; it is, however, an important component of enhancing the success of the program.

There are three distinct components of the Integrative Movement System Corrective Exercise Strategy™: release, activation, and integration.

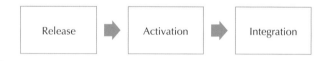

Integrative Movement System Corrective Exercise Strategy™ (Osar 2015).

Release

The first component of the strategy is to release the region in which the individual has restrictions that are preventing them from accessing the ideal muscles and/or movement patterns. Myofascial restrictions, adhesions following trauma, and scar tissue secondary to surgery can create fascial restrictions, loss of optimal tissue gliding, muscle inhibition, and joint restrictions. Independently, or in combination, these can lead to non-optimal postural and movement habits.

Release includes self-myofascial release (using myofascial tools), manual therapy, and breathing.

Clinically, Mindful Release™ is an extremely effective technique to help patients and clients "release" their chronic gripping strategy. Similar to how one cannot stretch a muscle that is consciously contracted, a muscle will not stretch where an individual is gripping for stability. For example, many individuals grip their hamstrings or superficial glutes, and when they attempt to stretch these muscles, they merely end up stretching the more flexible structures—such as their lumbar erectors. Mindful Release™ focuses an individual's attention on where they are over-contracting or gripping for stability (of which they are commonly not aware). Next they are cued to lightly isometrically contract and then slowly "release," "let go," and/or "lengthen" the muscle.

For a demonstration of Mindful Release, visit the website www.IIHFE.com/the-psoas-solution.

For many individuals with chronic tightness or discomfort, it is much more important to teach them where to stop gripping than to teach them how to activate a particular muscle or movement.

Activation

Muscle inhibition is weakness that occurs when the nervous system is unable to contract a muscle at its full physiological capacity. It can result from:

- *Reciprocal inhibition*: inhibition created by overactivity in antagonistic muscles.
- *Injury* (acute or repetitive): injury can lead to both local and global muscle inhibition.
- *Arthrogenic inhibition*: muscle inhibition that is created as a result of altered joint position and/or motion causing altered proprioception and therefore muscle contractibility.
- *Trigger points*: hyperirritable bands of contracted muscles that can decrease the overall force of a muscle contraction, and often contribute to early muscle fatigue during activity (Page et al. 2010).

- *Pseudoparesis*: as described by Janda, a type of muscle inhibition related to a neuroreflexive pattern that causes general hypotonus of a muscle, decreased strength on manual muscle testing, and delayed muscle onset, which results in synergist dominance (Page et al. 2010).
- *Deafferentation*: the reception of decreased sensory information from the peripheral neuromuscular receptors (proprioceptors), resulting in local and even distal losses in muscle strength (Page et al. 2010).
- *Fatigue*: includes overall general fatigue from lack of adequate sleep as well as from overusing a muscle during daily life, occupations, and particularly exercise, which can create and perpetuate temporary and even more long-term muscle inhibition issues.
- *Stretch weakness*: muscle inhibition that occurs secondarily to maintaining a muscle in a prolonged (chronic) overstretched position.
- *Tight weakness*: muscle inhibition that occurs secondarily to maintaining a muscle in a prolonged (chronic) shortened position.
- *Surgery*: clinical experience has demonstrated that many orthopedic surgeries, including minimally invasive procedures, creates a level of muscle inhibition, both locally in the muscles that were directly affected by the surgery, and globally when the muscles involve the abdominal wall, pelvic floor, spine, or to joint structures. Surgery likely results in both pseudoparesis and deafferentation which contributes to muscle inhibition.

Whether a muscle is inhibited or not should never be determined solely on the basis of postural evaluations and/or preconceived notions. The primary methods for detecting muscle inhibition include: manual muscle testing; palpation of the muscles involved (tissue quality, tone, etc.); and muscle timing and sequencing (which muscles fire first and/or the most). The cumulative outputs of each of these evaluative methods should be taken into consideration when determining muscle inhibition.

Facilitatory techniques (strategies to improve muscle activation)—such as visualization (mindful awareness and conscious attention), isometric contraction, palpation, and breathing—are an important part of the Integrative Movement System Corrective Exercise Strategy™ in restoring more optimal muscle activity in the presence of muscle inhibition. Many of these strategies have been demonstrated throughout this book.

Integration

Once the myofascial restrictions and/or gripping issues have been addressed, the individual must be taught how to integrate the newly acquired range of motion, alignment, breathing, and/or control strategy into the fundamental movement patterns (squatting, lunging, bending, rotating, pushing, pulling, and gait). This step is crucial in changing long-term postural and movement habits; if it is neglected, the individual's nervous system will often revert to its original non-optimal habit state.

Where corrective exercise approaches tend to fall short is when the clinician or fitness professional does not incorporate the changes gained through corrective exercise (range of motion, muscle activation, strength, improved breathing, postural/movement awareness, cuing, etc.) into the fundamental movement patterns. Hence, when the individual does not improve or demonstrate specific objective improvement after a period of performing "corrective" work, corrective exercise is abandoned because it failed to work. Corrective exercise did not fail; it is far more likely that it was the approach that failed.

With an understanding of what corrective exercise is, it is also important to understand what corrective exercise is not. Corrective exercise is not:

- a fix for an individual's postural dysfunction, muscle imbalances, and/or pain;

- a method for making individuals stand or sit with "perfect" posture or do their exercises in a "perfect" way;
- a group of remedial exercises that an individual performs to undo the effects of performing inappropriate exercises (i.e. the individual has performed exercises in which they cannot maintain their alignment, breathing, and control);
- a diagnosis or substitute for a thorough evaluation by a qualified health care professional;
- a substitute for a well-designed integrative strength training program.

Used judiciously, corrective exercise is an important part of an overall training strategy, designed to evaluate a client or patient as an individual and provide them with a valuable option for successfully addressing their issues, while working toward their functional goals. Corrective exercise should therefore encourage and not deter from improving strength, mobility, speed, endurance, or any other objective outcome. Essentially, corrective exercise helps to remove the barriers that prevent an individual from achieving their goals. Corrective exercise can and should be seamlessly incorporated into a comprehensive strength training program, so that the practitioner effectively helps any clients or patients (who have been struggling with chronic postural and/or movement issues) to safely and effectively accomplish their individual health and fitness goals.

This book contains many of the corrective exercise strategies used clinically to help individuals who are dealing with chronic posture and movement issues that are inhibiting them from performing at a level that they would like and/or need.

For more information on incorporating corrective exercise into your current programs, see Osar (2012) and check out the Integrative Corrective Exercise Approach™ website (http://integrativecorrectiveexercisespecialist.com).

Glossary

Agonists

Muscles that work together to produce a desire result. Generally, the muscles involved have similar functions on a particular joint. Example: the psoas and rectus femoris are agonists, because both muscles flex the hip; the gluteus maximus and hamstrings are agonists, because they both extend the hip.

Antagonists

Muscles that oppose the action of other muscles. Example: because the hip flexors flex the hip, and the hip extensors extend the hip, these two muscle groups are considered antagonists.

Activation

The facilitating or encouraging of conscious muscular activity. Also refers to facilitating more optimal muscular activity in an inhibited muscle.

Axis of Rotation

An imaginary line perpendicular to the plane of motion, about which a joint rotates. Joint centration helps maintain an optimal axis of rotation.

Centration

A theoretical position where the joint is optimally aligned and controlled. Each joint complex has a position in which the articular surfaces are best aligned for loading, and there is optimal myofascial control to support the joint during a specific activity.

Closed-chain Motion

The motion of a series of successively arranged joints, where the distal end of the segment is fixed to the floor or to an object. Example: a squatting or lunging pattern in which the foot is fixed on the ground and can therefore exert influence over the proximal segments of the kinetic chain.

Concentric Contraction

A contraction where the muscle shortens and its origin and insertion come closer together. Generally, contractions of this type are involved in creating and/or accelerating joint motion.

Control

(Also referred to as *motor control*.) The neuromuscular ability to maintain the most optimal and desired joint position and motion during a given activity. *Optimal control* promotes the most ideal or efficient posture and movement strategy, and potentially reduces the risk of injury. *Non-optimal control* refers to a less than ideal or inefficient posture and movement strategy, which increases the potential for overloading joints and soft tissues, and the risk of incurring a cumulative or repetitive injury.

Corrective Exercise

A specific approach that utilizes soft tissue release (manual or self-myofascial release) and specific exercises aimed at producing a more optimal or desirable outcome in posture and/or movement. Strategies to restore and/or maintain optimal alignment, breathing, and control form the basis of the Integrative Movement System Corrective Exercise Strategy™.

Deep Myofascial System (DMS)

The deep to intermediate layers of muscles and their investing fascia. The DMS is responsible for segmental stabilization, which provides specific joint control during posture and movement. The system features feedforward activation, which centrates a joint prior to movement. (See also Superficial Myofascial System.)

Dissociation

The ability to move one bony segment of a joint independently of its adjoining bony segment. Example: one must be able to dissociate or move the femoral head independently of the pelvis in open-chain motion, and also be able to dissociate the pelvis from femoral head motion in closed-chain motion. The loss of optimal joint dissociation leads to compensatory motion at one or more distal joint segments.

Distal

Furthest away from the center of the body.

Eccentric Contraction

A contraction where a muscle lengthens and its origin and insertion move further apart. Generally, contractions of this type are involved with slowing or stopping a motion, to prevent overstretching of the tissues on one side of a joint and over-compression on the opposite side.

Facilitation

The increasing of conscious muscle activity, generally in an inhibited muscle. Visualization,

isometric contractions, palpation, and breathing are methods used within the Integrative Movement System Corrective Exercise Strategy™ for facilitating desired muscle activity.

Fascia

Highly specialized connective tissue containing both sensory and contractile elements. Fascia surrounds and/or connects to most tissues in the body, including muscles, tendons, ligaments, and joint capsules, thereby providing support to these regions. Many muscles are fascially connected to each other, and so they can have an impact beyond the area in which they are physically located. Example: the psoas is fascially connected to the diaphragm as well as to the pelvic floor, and can thus have a direct impact on breathing and pelvic stability.

Feedforward

Central nervous system mediated control, which creates activation or contraction of the deep muscles, to provide joint stabilization just prior to movement. The loss of feedforward muscle activation has been noted in individuals experiencing chronic low back, pelvic, and neck pain, compared with individuals without pain.

Functional Synergists

Opposing muscles that work together to provide joint control and/or movement. Because these muscles have an opposing action to each other (and hence are generally categorized as *antagonists*), when working together they are called *functional synergists* to differentiate them from muscles that always work together (see Synergists). Example: the psoas and gluteus maximus are generally considered antagonists, as the former is a hip extensor and the latter is a hip flexor; however, they must function together in order to provide control of the femoral head in the acetabulum during functional activity.

Fundamental Movement Patterns

The movement patterns essential to life, sports, and occupations. Virtually all human movement can be broken down into fundamental movement patterns, including squatting, lunging, bending, rotating, pushing, pulling, and balance/gait. The goal of corrective and functional exercise is to provide an environment for improving an individual's efficiency in performing the fundamental movement patterns.

Gripping

The over-activation or over-contraction of a particular muscle to provide joint stability or control. This overactivity often leads to the loss of joint centration and/or over-compression of the joints around the area of overactivity. Common muscles involved in gripping that affects the spine or hips include the superficial erector spinae, superficial abdominals, superficial gluteus maximus, and superficial hip flexors (e.g. rectus femoris and tensor fasciae latae).

Inhibition

Refers (in the context of this book) to the inability to optimally activate a neurologically intact muscle, as needed for postural support or movement. Generally, this type of muscle inhibition is present in the absence of a true underlying neurological pathology. (See Appendix VII on corrective exercise for more on muscle inhibition.) Muscle inhibition is detected through muscle testing as taught in Applied Kinesiology (George Goodheart, DC) or Clinical Kinesiology (Alan Beardall, DC). An inhibited muscle will generally test strong when tested in a lengthened position, but weak when tested in the shortened position. By utilizing a muscle activation strategy (such as an isometric contraction with joint centration, origin-insertion muscle palpation, and/or breathing), muscle strength (the ability to contract on demand) can be restored.

Isometric Contraction

A contraction where there is no change in the length of the muscle. Generally, isometric contractions are involved in stabilizing a joint. Some two-joint muscles (e.g. rectus femoris and hamstrings) will lengthen at one end and shorten at the other, so that there is no net change in the length of the muscle; this is sometimes referred to as a *pseudo-isometric contraction*.

Kinetic Chain

A series of successively arranged joints, connected both physically and neurally. Example: the *lower kinetic chain* includes the foot, ankle, knee, and hip; the hand, wrist, elbow, and shoulder constitute the *upper kinetic chain*.

Micro-breaks

Short (micro-) and regular breaks (purposeful interruptions) from repetitive positions or work, designed to reset an individual's postural, breathing, and/or movement strategy. During micro-breaks, the focus is generally on the individual's alignment, breathing, or control strategy that addresses the most important driver of their issue.

Mindful Release™

A specific release technique taught as part of the Corrective Exercise Strategy™ aimed at releasing chronic myofascial holding (gripping) patterns. Mindful Release™ brings one's conscious awareness to regions of unconscious myofascial contraction, thereby assisting the individual to "let go" of those holding patterns. The strategy generally involves using a contract–relax strategy that is coordinated with breathing, while cuing to "release," "lengthen," or "let go" of the region(s) of myofascial contraction.

Mindfulness

Bringing conscious awareness and deliberate attention to a region of one's body or to one's posture or movement, to create a more optimal or desirable outcome. Mindful exercise is an important component in changing chronic postural and movement habits, as well as in adopting a more optimal strategy.

Open-chain Motion

Motion of a series of successively arranged joints, where the distal end of the segment is not fixed to the floor or to an object, and can move freely. Example: a seated leg-extension or lying leg-curl machine, where the foot is not locked onto the ground and therefore does not technically influence what happens at the more proximal joints of the kinetic chain.

Osteoarthritis

(Also referred to as *degenerative joint disease—DJD*). A gradual and usually progressive wear and tear on the joints, resulting in diminished cartilage, excessive bone growth, and at times pain. Generally, osteoarthritis is related to an individual's posture and movement habits, as well as to previous injuries and surgeries. It is a lifestyle issue and not a genetic or hereditary issue like other types of autoimmune arthritis such as rheumatoid.

Prone

Lying in a face-down position.

Proximal

Closest to the center of the body.

Quadruped

Supporting the body on the hands or forearms and knees (all-fours).

Release

Soft tissue work (myofascial release or similar strategy) that aims to release myofascial contractions. It also includes the ability to communicate with the nervous system to relax, or "let go," of chronic myofascial holding (gripping) patterns. (See also Mindful Release™.)

Spinal Stenosis

A narrowing (stenosis) of the spinal canal where the spinal cord runs through the vertebrae, or where the intervertebral canal narrows around the region where the nerve roots exit from the spinal cord into the periphery. Spinal stenosis can result in radicular symptoms (nerve-type sensations, such as numbness, tingling, or electrical type pain) and/or can affect muscle function in the extremities.

Strategy

Coordination of the neuromuscular system in order to produce a specific response. The goal of assessments is to identify an individual's strategy for posture and movement. The goal of a corrective exercise strategy is to help the individual develop a more optimal and efficient strategy for posture and movement, to enhance function and to reduce the potential for injury.

Superficial Myofascial System (SMS)

Intermediate to superficial layers of muscles and their investing fascia. The general role of the SMS is to produce gross (non-specific) joint stabilization and movement. (See also Deep Myofascial System.)

Supine

Lying in a face-up position.

Syndromes

A collection of related pathological signs and symptoms. Example: a decrease in hip range of motion, anterior hip pain during hip range of motion, and deep hip pain during the hip impingement test are signs and symptoms of hip impingement syndrome.

Synergists

Muscles that work together to provide joint control and/or movement. (See also Functional Synergists.)

System

A group of structures with coordinated activities, working collectively to achieve the same general function in the body. Example: the neuromusculoskeletal system consists of the nervous, muscular (including fascia, ligaments, and related connective tissue), and skeletal systems. The neuromuscular fascial system collectively contributes to posture, stability, and movement.

Bibliography

General

Andersson, E., Oddsson, L., Grundstrom, H., and Thorstensson, A. 1995. The role of the psoas and iliacus muscles for stability and movement of the lumbar spine, pelvis and hip. *Scandanavian Journal of Medicine and Science in Sports* 5, 10–16.

Barker, K.L., Shamley, D.R., and Jackson, D. 2004. Changes in the cross-sectional area of multifidus and psoas in patients with unilateral back pain. *Spine* 29(22), E515–E519.

Benz, A., Winkelman, N., Porter, J., and Nimphius, S. 2016. Coaching instructions and cues for enhancing sprint performance. *Strength & Conditioning Journal* 38(1), 1–11.

Blankenbaker, D.G., Tuite, M.J., Keene, J.S., and Munez del Rio, A. 2012. Labral injuries due to iliopsoas impingement: Can they be diagnosed on MR arthrography? *American Journal of Radiology* 199, 894–900.

Bogduk, N. 2005. *Clinical Anatomy of the Lumbar Spine and Sacrum*, 4th edn. Elsevier: New York.

Bordoni, B. and Marelli, F. 2016. Failed back surgery syndrome: review and new hypotheses. *Journal of Pain Research* 9, 17–22.

Bordoni, B. and Zanier, E. 2013. Anatomic connections of the diaphragm: Influence of respiration on the body system. *Journal of Multidisciplinary Healthcare* 3(6), 281–291.

Brandenburg, J.B., Kapron, A.L., Wylie, J.D., Wilkinson, B.G., Maak, T.G., Gonzalez, C.D., and Aoki, S.K. 2016. The functional and structural outcomes of arthroscopic iliopsoas release. *American Journal of Sports Medicine* 44(5), 1286–1291.

Capson, A.C., Nashed, J., and McClean, L. 2011. The Role of lumbopelvic posture in pelvic floor muscle activation in continent women. *Journal of Electromyographic Kinesiology* 21(1), 166–167.

Carrière, B. 2002. *Fitness for the Pelvic Floor*. Thieme: Stuttgart, Germany.

Casale, M., Sabatino, L., Moffa, A., Capuano, F., Luccarelli, V., Vitali, M., Ribolsi, M., Cicala, M., and Salvinelli, F. 2016. Breathing training on lower esophageal sphincter as a complementary treatment of gastroesophageal reflux disease (GERD): A systematic review. *European Review of Medical and Pharmacological Science* 20(21), 4547–4552.

Chaitow, L., Bradley, D., and Gilbert, C. 2014. *Recognizing and Treating Breathing Disorders,* 2nd edn. Elsevier: New York.

Cleveland Clinic Foundation 2014. What are vital signs? (<https://my.clevelandclinic.org/health/diagnostics/hic_Vital_Signs> Accessed January 23, 2016).

Dangaria, T.R. and Naesh, O. 1998. Changes in cross-sectional area of psoas major muscle in unilateral sciatica caused by disc herniation. *Spine* 23(8), 928–931.

Danneels, L.A., Vanderstraeten, G.G., Cambier, D.C., Witvrouw, E.E., and De Cuyper, H.J. 2000. CT imaging of trunk muscles in chronic low back pain patients and healthy control subjects. *European Spine Journal* 9, 266–272.

di Vico, R., Ardigo, L.C., Salernitano, G., Chamari, K., and Pudulo, J. 2013. The acute effect of the tongue position in the mouth on knee isokinetic test performance: A highly surprising pilot study. *Muscles Ligaments Tendons Journal* 3(4), 318–323.

Dobbs, M.B., Gordon, J.E., Luhmann, S.J., Szymanski, D.A., and Schoenecker, P.L. 2002. Surgical correction of the snapping iliopsoas tendon in adolescents. *American Journal of Bone and Joint Surgery* 84-A(3), 420–424.

Dooley, P.J. 2008. Femoroacetabular impingement syndrome. *Canadian Family Physician* 54, 42–47.

Dostal, W.F., Soderberg, G.L., and Andrews, J.G. 1986. Actions of hip muscles. *Physical Therapy* 66, 351–359.

FitzGordon, J. 2013. *Psoas Release Party!* FitzGordon Method Books: Lexington, KY.

Fortin, M. and Macedo, L.G. 2013. Multifidus and paraspinal muscle group cross-sectional areas of patients with low back pain and control patients: A systematic review with focus on blinding. *Physical Therapy* 93(7), 873–888.

Franklin, E. 1996. *Dynamic Alignment Through Imagery.* Human Kinetics: Champaign, IL.

Franklin, E. 2004. *Conditioning for Dance: Training for Peak Performance in All Dance Forms.* Human Kinetics: Champaign, IL.

Franklin, E. 2011. *The Psoas: Integrating Your Inner Core.* OPTP: Minneapolis, MN.

Garrison, J.C., Osler, M.T., and Singleton, S.B. 2007. Rehabilitation after arthroscopy of an acetabular labral tear. *North American Journal of Sports Physical Therapy* 2(4), 241–250.

Gibbons, S.G.T. 2005a. Integrating the psoas major and deep sacral gluteus maximus muscles into the lumbar cylinder model. *Proceedings of "The Spine": World Congress on Manual Therapy.* 7–9th October, Rome, Italy.

Gibbons, S.G.T. 2005b. *Assessment & Rehabilitation of the Stability Function of the Psoas Major and the Deep Sacral Gluteus Maximus Muscles.* Kinetic Control: Ludlow, UK.

Gibbons, S.G.T. 2007. Assessment and rehabilitation of the stability function of psoas major. *Manuelle Therapie* 11, 177–187.

Gibbons, S.G.T., Comerford, M.J., and Emerson, P.L. 2002. Rehabilitation of the stability function of psoas major. *Orthopaedic Division Review*, Jan/Feb, 9–16.

Gildea, J.E., VanDen, H.W., Hides, J.A., and Hodges, P.W. 2015. Trunk dynamics are impaired in ballet dancers with back pain but improve with imagery. *Medicine and Science in Sports and Exercise* 47(8), 1665–1671.

Gruber, H.E., Rhyne, A.L., Hansen, K.J., Phillips, R.C., Hoelscher, G.L., Ingram, J.A. and Hanley, E.N.Jr. 2015. Deleterious effects of discography radiocontrast solution on human annulus cell in vitro: changes in cell viability, proliferation, and apoptosis in exposed cells. *Spine* 12(4), 329–335.

Hagins, M., Pietrek, M.D., Sheikhzadeh, A., Nordin, M., and Axen, K. 2004. The effects of breath control on intra-abdominal pressure during lifting tasks. *Spine* 29(4), 464–469.

Hall, L., Tsao, H., MacDonald, D., Coppieters, M., and Hodges, P.W. 2009. Immediate effects of co-contraction training on motor control of the trunk muscles in people with recurrent low back pain. *Journal of Electromyographic Kinesiology* 19(5), 763–773.

Hides, J.A. and Stanton, W.R. 2014. Can motor control training lower the risk of injury for professional football players? *Medicine and Science in Sports and Exercise* 46(4), 762–768.

Hides, J.A., Endicott, T., Mendis, M.D., and Stanton, W.R. 2016. The effect of motor control training on abdominal muscle contraction during simulated weight bearing in elite cricketers. *Physical Therapy in Sport* 20, 26–31.

Hides, J., Stanton, W., McMahon, S., Sims, K., and Richardson, C. 2008, Effect of stabilization training on multifidus muscle cross-sectional area among young elite cricketers with low back pain. *Journal of Orthopaedic & Sports Physical Therapy* 38(3), 101–112.

Hides, J.A., Stanton, W.R., Mendis, M.D., Gildea, J., and Sexton, M.J. 2012. Effect of motor control training on muscle size and football games missed from injury. *Medicine and Science in Sports and Exercise* 44(6), 1141–1149.

Hodges, P.W., Cholewicki, J., and van Dieen, J. 2013. *Spinal Control: The Rehabilitation of Back Pain*. Churchill Livingstone Elsevier: Edinburgh, UK.

Hodges, P.W., Sapsford, R., and Pengel, L.H. 2007. Postural and respiratory functions of the pelvic floor muscles. *Neurology Urodynamics* 26(3), 362–371.

Hodges, P.W., Moseley, G.L., Gabrielsson, A., and Gandevia, S.C. 2003. Experimental muscle pain changes feedforward postural responses of the trunk muscles. *Experimental Brain Research* 151(2), 262–271.

Hu, H., Meijer, O.G., van Dieen, J.H., Hodges, P.W., Bruijn, S.M., Strijers, R.L., Nanayakkara, W.B., van Royen, B.J., Wu, W.H., and Xia, C. 2011. Is the psoas a hip flexor in the active straight leg raise? *European Spine Journal* 20, 759–765.

Hwang, D.S., Hwang, J.M., Kim, P.S., Rhee, S.M., Park, S.H., Kang, S.Y., and Ha, Y.C. 2015. Arthroscopic treatment of symptomatic internal snapping hip with combined pathologies. *Clinics in Orthopedic Surgery* 7, 158–163.

Kim, J.W., Kang, M.H., and Oh, J.S. 2014. Patients with low back pain demonstrate increased activity of the posterior oblique sling muscle during prone hip extension. *American Academy of Physical Medicine and Rehabilitation* 6, 400–405.

Kim, W.H., Lee, S.H., and Lee, D.Y. 2011. Changes in the cross-sectional area of multifidus and psoas in unilateral sciatic caused by lumbar disc herniation. *Journal of Korean Neurosurgery Society* 50, 201–204.

Koch, L. 1997. *The Psoas Book*, 2nd edn. Guinea Pig Publications: Felton, CA.

Kolar, P. et al. 2013. *Clinical Rehabilitation*. Alena Kobesova: K. Vapence 16, Praha 5.

Kuhlman, G.S. and Domb, B.G. 2009. Hip impingement: Identifying and treating a common cause of hip pain. *American Family Physician* 80(12), 1429–1434.

Lamoth, C.J.C., Meijer, O.G., Daffertshofer, A., Wuisman, P.I.J.M., and Beek, P.J. 2006. Effects of chronic low back pain on trunk coordination and back muscle activity during walking: Changes in motor control. *European Spine Journal* 15, 23–40.

Lee, D. 2003. *The Thorax: An Integrated Approach*, 2nd edn. Diane G. Lee Physiotherapist Corp: White Rock, BC.

Lee, D. 2012. *The Pelvic Girdle: An Approach to the Examination and Treatment of the Lumbopelvic-hip Region*, 4th edn. Churchill Livingstone: Edinburgh.

Lee, D. and Lee, L.J. 2014. *Treating the Whole Person—The Integrated Systems Model for Pain & Disability*. Course handouts. Vancouver, BC.

Lewis C.A., Sahrmann, S.A., Moran, D.W. 2007. Anterior hip joint forces increases with hip extension, decreased gluteal force, or decreased iliopsoas force. *Journal of Biomechanics* 40, 3725–3731.

Massery, M. 2006. The patient with multi-system impairments affecting breathing mechanics and motor control. In: Frownfelter, D. and Dean, E., eds. *Cardiovascular and Pulmonary Physical Therapy Evidence and Practice*, 4th edn. Mosby & Elsevier Health Sciences: St. Louis, MO.

Mendis, M.D. and Hides, J.A. 2016. Effect of motor control training on hip muscles in elite football players with and without low back pain. *Journal of Science in Medicine and Sport* 19(11), 866–871.

Michaud, T. 2011. *Human Locomotion*. Newton Biomechanics: Newton, MA.

McGill, S. 2004. *Ultimate Back Fitness and Performance.* Wabuno: Waterloo, Ontario.

McGill, S. 2007. *Low Back Disorders: Evidence-based Prevention and Rehabilitation*, 2nd edn. Human Kinetics: Champaign, IL.

Myers, T.W. 2014. *Anatomy Trains.* Churchill Livingstone: Edinburgh.

Nelson, I.R. and Keene, J.S. 2014. Results of labral-level arthroscopic iliopsoas tenotomies for the treatment of labral impingement. *Arthroscopy* 30(6), 688–694.

Neumann, D.A. and Garceau, L.R. 2014. A proposed novel function of the psoas minor revealed through cadaver dissection. *Clinical Anatomy* 28(2), 242–252.

Niemelainen, R., Briand, M.M., and Battie, M.C. 2011. Substantial asymmetry in paraspinal muscle cross-sectional area in healthy adults questions its value as a marker of low back pain and pathology. *Spine* 36(25), 2152–2157.

Nygaard, I.E., Thompson, F.L., Svengalis, S.L., and Albright, J.P. 1994. Urinary incontinence in elite nulliparous athletes. *Obstetrics Gynecology* 84(2), 183–187.

Osar, E. 2012. *Corrective Exercise Solutions to Common Hip and Shoulder Dysfunction*. Lotus Publishing: Chichester, UK.

Osar, E. 2015. *Integrative Movement Systems Mastery Series: The Thoracopelvic Canister*. Course handouts. Chicago, IL.

Osar, E. and Bussard, M. 2016. *Functional Anatomy of the Pilates Core*. Lotus Publishing: Chichester, UK.

Paalanne, N. Niinimaki, J., Karppinen, J., Taimela, S., Mutanen, P., Takatalo, J., Korpelainen, R., and Tervonen, O. 2011. Assessment of association between low back pain and paraspinal muscle atrophy using magnetic resonance imaging: a population-based study among young adults. *Spine* 36(23), 1961–1968.

Page, P., Frank, C.C., and Lardner, R. 2010. *Assessment and Treatment of Muscle Imbalance: the Janda Approach*. Human Kinetics: Champaign, IL.

Penning, L. 2000. Psoas muscle and lumbar spine stability: a concept uniting existing controversies. *European Spine Journal* 9, 577–585.

Penning, L. 2002. Spine stabilization by psoas muscle during walking and running. *European Spine Journal* 11, 89–90.

Ploumis, A., Michailidis, N., Christodoulou, P., Kalaitzoglou, I., Gouvas, G., and Beris, A. Ipsilateral atrophy of paraspinal and psoas muscle in unilateral back pain patients with nonsegmental degenerative disc disease. *British Journal of Radiology* 84(100), 709–713.

Poswiatia, A., Socha, T., and Opara, J. 2014. Prevalence of stress urinary incontinence in elite female endurance athletes. *Journal of Human Kinetics* 44, 91–96.

Retchford, T.H., Crossley, K.M., Grimaldi, A., Kemp, J.L., Cowan, S.M. 2013. Can local muscles augment stability in the hip? A narrative literature review. *Journal of Musculoskeletal Neuronal Interaction* 13(1), 1–12.

Richardson, C., Hides, J., and Hodges, P.W. 2004. *Therapeutic Exercise for Lumbopelvic Stabilization: a Motor Control Approach for the Treatment and Prevention of Low Back Pain*, 2nd edn. Churchill Livingstone: Edinburgh.

Sackett, D.L., Rosenburg, W.M.C., Muir Gray, J.A., Haynes, R. B., and Richardson, W.S. 1996. Evidence-based medicine: What it is and what it isn't. *British Medical Journal* 312, 71.

Sahrmann, S. 2002. *Diagnosis and Treatment of Movement Impairment Syndromes*. Mosby: St. Louis, MO.

Sajko, S. and Stuber, K. 2009. Psoas Major: A case report and review of its anatomy, biomechanics, and clinical implications. *Journal of the Canadian Chiropractic Association* 53(4), 311–318.

Salata, M.J., Gibbs, A.E., and Sekiya, J.K. 2010. A systemic reviw of clinical outcomes in patients undergoing meniscectomy. *American Journal of Sports Medicine* 38(9), 1907–1916.

Sapsford, R.R., Richardson, C.A., Maher, C.F., and Hodges, P.W. 2008. Pelvic floor muscle activity in different sitting postures in continent and incontinent women. *Archives of Physical Medicine and Rehabilitation* 89(9), 1741–1747.

Sapsford, R.R., Hodges, P.W., Richardson, C.A., Cooper, D.H., Markwell, S.J., and Jull, G.A. 2001. Co-activation of the abdominal and pelvic floor muscles during voluntary exercises. *Neurologic Urodynamics* 20(1), 31–42.

Saragiotto, B.T., Maher, C.G., Yamato, T.P., Costa, L.O., Menezes Costa, L.C., Ostelo, R.W., and Macedo, L.G. 2016. Motor control exercise for chronic non-specific low-back pain. *Cochrane Database Systemic Review* 41(16), 1284–1291.

Schuster, C., Hilfiker, R., Amft, O., Schneidhauer, A., Andrews, B., Butler, J., Kischka, U., and Ettlin, T. 2011. Best practice for motor imagery: A systematic literature review on motor imagery training elements in five different disciplines. *British Medical Journal* 9(75), 1–35.

Seongho, K., Hyungguen, K., and Jaeyeop, C. 2014. Effects of spinal stabilization exercise on the cross-sectional areas of the lumbar multifidus and psoas major muscles, pain intensity, and lumbar muscle strength of patients with degenerative disc disease. *Journal of Physical Therapy Science* 26(4), 579–582.

Smith, D. 2004. Female pelvic floor health. *Journal of Wound Ostomy and Continence Nursing* 31(3), 137.

Smith, M.D., Coppieters, M.W., and Hodges, P.W. 2008. Is balance different in women with and without stress urinary incontinence? *Neurologic Urodynamics* 27(1), 71–78.

Stecco C. 2015. *Functional Atlas of the Human Fascial System*. Churchill Livingstone, Elsevier: New York.

Steffens, D., Maher, C.G., Pereira, L.S., Stevens, M.L., Oliveira, V.C., Chapple, M., Teixeira-Salmela, L.F., and Hancock, M.J. 2016. Prevention of low back pain: A systematic review and meta-analysis. *Journal of the American Medical Association Internal Medicine* 11, 1–10.

Sullivan, M.S. 1989. Back support mechanisms during manual lifting. *Physical Therapy* 69, 38–45.

Taylor, G.R. and Clarke, N.M.P. 1995. Surgical release of the "snapping hip tendon." *The Journal of Bone and Joint Surgery* 77-B, 881–883.

Tsao, H. and Hodges, P.W. 2007. Immediate changes in feedforward postural adjustments following voluntary motor training. *Experimental Brain Research* 181(4), 537–546.

Tsao, H. and Hodges, P.W. 2008. Persistence of improvements in postural strategies following motor control training in people with recurrent low back pain. *Journal of Electromyographic Kinesiology* 18(4), 559–567.

Thyssen, H.H., Clevin, L., Olesen, S., and Lose, G. 2002. Urinary incontinence in elite female athletes and dancers. *International Urogynecology Journal* 13(1), 15–17.

Umphred, D.A. 2007. *Neurological Rehabilitation*, 5th edn. Mosby Elsevier: St. Louis, MO.

Vleeming, A. 2012. *Understanding the diagnostics and treatment of the lumbopelvic spine*. Course handouts. Chicago, IL.

Vostatek, P., Novák, D., Rychnovský, T., and Rychnovská, S. 2013. Diaphragm postural function analysis using magnetic resonance imaging. *PLOS ONE* 8(3), 1–13.

Yazbek, P.M., Ovanessian, V., Martin, R.L., and Fukuda, T.Y. 2011. Nonsurgical treatment of acetabular labrum tears: A case series. *Journal of Orthopedic and Sports Physical Therapy* 41(5), 346–353.

Yoon, T.L., Kim, K.S., Cynn, and H.S. 2014. Slow expiration reduces sternocleidomastoid activity and increases transversus abdominis and internal oblique muscle activity during abdominal curl-up. *Journal of Electromyographic Kinesiology* 24(2), 228–232.

Manual Muscle Testing

Beardall, A.G. 1982. *Clinical Kinesiology Instruction Manual*. A.G. Beardall, D.C., Lake: Oswego, OR.

Beardall, A.G. 1983. *Clinical Kinesiology Vol IV: Muscles of the Upper Extremities, Shoulder, Forearm, and Hand*. Lake Oswego, OR.

Beardall, A.G. 1985. *Clinical Kinesiology Vol V: Muscles of the Lower Extremities, Calf, and Foot*. Lake Oswego, OR.

Beardall, A.G. and Beardall C.A. 2006a. *Clinical Kinesiology Vol I: Low Back and Abdomen*. Woodburn, OR.

Beardall, A.G. and Beardall C.A.: 2006b. *Clinical Kinesiology Vol II: Pelvis and Thigh*. Woodburn, OR.

Beardall, A.G. and Beardall C.A.: 2006c. *Clinical Kinesiology Vol III: TMJ, Hyoid, and Other Cervical Muscles and Cranial Manipulation*. Woodburn, OR.

Buhler, C. 2004. *The Evaluation and Treatment of Low Back & Abdomen*. Course handouts. Kaysville, UT.

Frost, R. 2002. *Applied Kinesiology: A Training Manual and Reference Book of Basic Principles and Practice*. North Atlantic: Berkeley, CA.

Kendall, F.P., McCreary, E.K., Provance, P.G., Rodgers, M.M., and Romani, W.A. 2005. *Muscles: Testing and Function with Posture and Pain*, 5th edn. Lippincott Williams & Wilkins: Baltimore, MD.

Walther, D.S. 2000. *Applied Kinesiology: Synopsis*, 2nd edn. Systems DC: Pueblo, CO.

Index